easy meal prep

SAVE TIME AND EAT HEALTHY
WITH OVER 75 RECIPES

ERIN ROMEO

ROCK POINT

This edition published in 2025 by Rock Point,
an imprint of The Quarto Group,
142 West 36th Street, 4th Floor,
New York, NY 10018, USA
(212) 779-4972
www.Quarto.com

First published in 2019 as *The Visual Guide to Easy Meal Prep* by Race Point Publishing, an imprint of The Quarto Group, 142 West 36th Street, 4th Floor, New York, NY 10018, USA.

Rock Point titles are also available at discount for retail, wholesale, promotional and bulk purchase. For details, contact the Special Sales Manager by email at specialsales@quarto.com or by mail at The Quarto Group, Attn: Special Sales Manager, 100 Cummings Center Suite, 265D, Beverly, MA 01915, USA.

10 9 8 7 6 5 4 3 2 1

ISBN: 978-1-57715-506-5

Library of Congress Cataloging-in-Publication Data

Names: Romeo, Erin, author.
Title: Easy meal prep : save time and eat healthy with over 75 recipes /
    Erin Romeo.
Description: New York, NY : Rock Point, 2025. | Includes index. | Summary:
    "Meal prep is essential for any diet. Easy Meal Prep will help you plan
    to eat for success"– Provided by publisher.
Identifiers: LCCN 2024027605 | ISBN 9781577155065 (paperback)
Subjects: LCSH: Quick and easy cooking. | Cooking (Natural foods) |
    Cooking–Planning. | LCGFT: Cookbooks.
Classification: LCC TX833.5 .R6557 2025 | DDC 641.5/12–dc23/eng/20240625
LC record available at https://lccn.loc.gov/2024027605

Publisher: Rage Kindelsperger
Creative Director: Laura Drew
Editorial Director: Erin Canning
Managing Editor: Cara Donaldson
Cover and Interior Design: Laura Klynstra
Food Photography: Alison Bickel Photography (except for the following pages
15, 30, 32, 40, 48, 52, 78, 100, 106, 109, 117, 118, 123, 126, 130, 134, 136 and 137)
Author Photography: Saleme Fayad

Printed in China

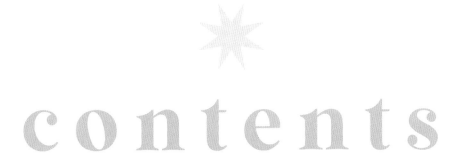

contents

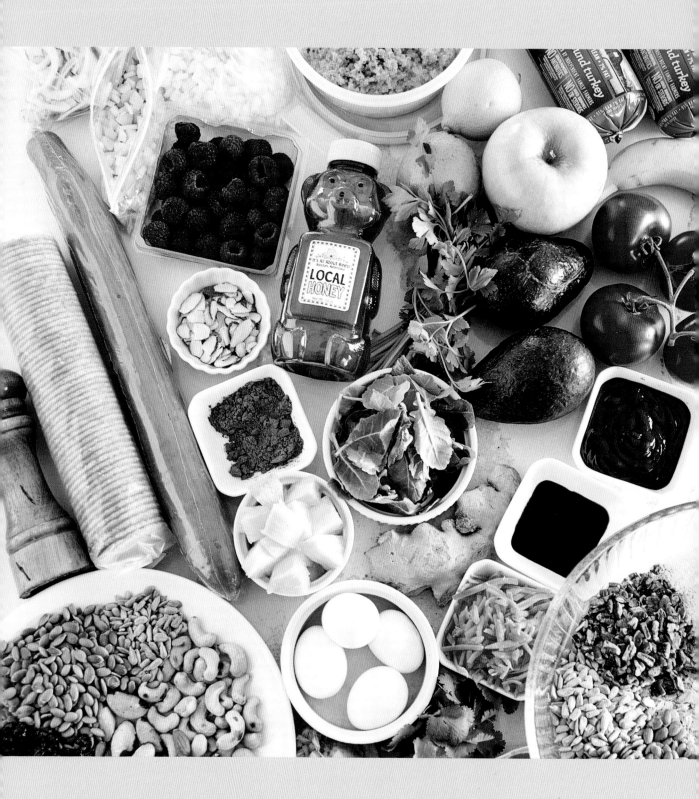

introduction

I'M SO GLAD YOU'RE HERE! If you have meal-prepped, attempted to meal-prep, or thought about meal prep before, you're in the right place. I've been teaching others my formula for meal prep and meal planning for over ten years in workshops and small groups, and I've also had (and still have) the pleasure of working with clients one-on-one as a nutrition coach. The one takeaway I've discovered from all my coaching is how valuable meal prep and planning is. Over the years, I have found that meal preparation is the most underutilized strategy for healthy eating. Period. If what you desire is real change, it's critical that you pay attention to the food you consume. Once you learn how to prepare them in easy, healthy, and convenient ways, you will wonder why you waited so long to incorporate this simple routine. Beyond the health benefits of meal prep, after just one week of doing it, my clients have raved about how it's changed everything for them, and how accomplished they feel at the end of a meal-prep session, when neatly placing their food-filled containers into the fridge. They also have said how great it is to grab their prepped food for work every day without spending time, effort, or energy on having to think about what to make or spend money on healthy takeout.

It has taken me years of prepping for myself and my family to create a system that works for the long term. My system is easy to follow, and anyone can do it. I fully trust that you, too, will benefit from this process and all the benefits that result from it. In fact, I know you will. I've had (and continue to have) clients from all over the world who share their successes with me. After reading comments time after time like, "It's a lot easier than I thought" or "I just follow your process and it's working!," I knew I had to collect and share what I was teaching. This is how my 5 Steps to Meal-Prep Success (page 8) was born.

The daily stress of deciding what to eat, cooking, and cleaning is behind you. Even if you haven't meal-prepped before, or think it will be overwhelming or complicated, you can and will do this! Whether you're starting small (lunches for your work week) or going for the big win (an entire week of meals and snacks), these five steps will have you on your way to meal-prep victory in no time.

WHAT IS MEAL PREP?

Simply put, "meal prep," or "food prep," is preparing several meals all at once through the acts of shopping, washing, cutting, cooking, and packaging. This practice has been around for a long time. In the past, food prep and batch cooking were most commonly seen in large families; they had no other choice but to prepare large quantities of food to ensure there was something for everyone to eat. Maybe this is what you think about when you hear the words "meal prep." More recently, meal prep has become popular in fitness and bodybuilding circles, where athletes haul around precisely portioned containers of food, consuming a certain number of calories a day to ensure peak performance. But for the purpose of this book, meal prep is the go-to method for people just like you and me, looking to live a healthier and more organized lifestyle. Whether you're interested in cooking for yourself, your significant other, or your entire family, adopting my meal-prep system is doable and life-changing. I know the term "life-changing" gets thrown around a lot. Recently, I was shopping, and the salesperson said, "This cable-knit sweater is life-changing." Really? I don't know about that, but what I do know is this: once you start meal prepping, your entire life will change for the better. The benefits of the simple act of meal preparation will trickle down into other parts of your life too.

WHY MEAL-PREP?

From my experience, most people explore the world of meal prep to experience the health benefits it provides. This is certainly what will happen once you incorporate my routine, but it's actually the unexpected benefits that amaze most people and what I love hearing about:

* You will regain hours in your day. I cannot emphasize this enough. You'll have more time each day to do the things you never had time to do. You'll have more time to relax, to learn something new, or fit in another healthy habit like daily exercise or meditation.

* You will eliminate the need to multitask as you prepare lunch or dinner.

* You'll be more present with the people around you. For those of you with children at home, that means no more bouncing back and forth between the kitchen and family room, watching the stove and helping with homework at the same time.

Picture the beginning of your day. Think about what it will be like to wake up each morning knowing your tasty and healthy breakfast is already waiting for you. Say goodbye to those frantic mornings of running out of your house, fighting traffic, and racing against the clock as you try to squeeze in a drive-through run for something to eat. The money and time you'll save each morning will add up quickly. The best part of my coaching is when these unexpected 12 benefits accumulate for my clients. We end up planning the ways they are going to use the money and time they've saved—anything from a date night to purchasing some new clothes to fit your slimmer waistline.

As much as meal prep is about getting organized and taking control of your overall health, the physical changes that are experienced are just as rewarding. When I hear my clients talk about the compliments and accolades they receive from their coworkers and friends because of their increased energy and weight loss, I can't help but join in their excitement. I bet you didn't think meal prep could be this transformative, did you? Well it is, and I want you to experience all of this too.

WHERE TO START?

The best part of meal prepping is that you get to direct it, by using my strategy and making it your own. Some people prep a week's worth of food in one day, while others organize two "mini preps" for a few days at a time. No matter which method you choose, food prepping is all about routine. And once you practice this new routine, it will become second nature to you. You'll develop an important healthy habit that will serve you for years to come.

Remember, although it might seem daunting at first, the routine I walk you through is tried and tested—all you need to do is follow it, step-by-step. As you become more comfortable with cook times, organization, and food combinations, you can tweak the routine to best suit your lifestyle. I commonly say, "It's not hard; it just takes practice." It's true. It's not hard to follow a meal-prep routine. All you need are three ingredients: a proven routine, some patience, and an open and willing attitude. I bring the first ingredient; I need you to bring the other two!

There have been numerous studies confirming that people who prepare meals at home are more likely to have healthier diets. This may seem like an obvious conclusion, but, as you know, it's easier said than done. Home-prepared meals are healthier, and when combined with a regular cooking routine, home-prepared meals lead to a healthier lifestyle that's sustainable for the long run. Cooking at home has another advantage: the cost factor. It's significantly less expensive to eat at home than to eat out (fast food and casual dining alike). So, why aren't we cooking at home all the time? I have listened to my clients, friends, and family repeatedly tell me that most people aren't cooking at home because they "don't have the time to do it." I, too, believed that I didn't have the time to prepare meals at home. It's only in hindsight that I can now honestly say that I don't have time not to meal-prep.

HOW LONG DOES IT TAKE?

The Organization for Economic Cooperation and Development (OECD) studied time spent on unpaid work in thirty-four countries and found that people spend an average of two hours and eight minutes per day on meal preparation and cleanup. Even if you only spend half the average time on these tasks, that's still seven to fourteen hours of washing, cutting, cooking, packing meals, and cleaning up every week. Whew, that's a lot of time! And that's time better spent doing other things you want to do (you know, those "things" you always say you wish you had more time to do).

I am so confident in the efficiency of my 5 Steps to Meal-Prep Success (page 8) that I can guarantee you will only need two to three hours, once per week, to reap the numerous rewards that meal prep offers. Granted, in the beginning, it may take you a little more time to learn a new routine and incorporate some rituals you may have never used before, but with a little practice and the easy-to-follow recipes found in this book, you'll be a meal-prep pro in no time. You will be well on your way to a fridge full of healthy meals and an even better you.

the five steps to meal-prep success

These are the exact five steps I've been using for years to prepare my own meals for the entire week in two to three hours, and it's the same system I teach my clients so they can achieve their goals. Following a prescribed set of steps to carry out any task is a surefire way to get the results you're looking for. This is especially true with meal prep. It can seem daunting in the beginning, but if you start small, prepping just three lunches or two dinners, you will build that prep muscle to a full week's worth of prep in a few hours, and you can say goodbye to daily cooking and cleaning and hello to nutritious, ready-to-eat meals.

Okay, so are you ready to start prepping?! The first thing I want you to do is take out your calendar and pick your prep day. If you are planning to prepare meals for the entire week, block out two to three hours, or three to four hours if you're new to meal prepping. As you become accustomed to the recipes and meal-prep rituals, it will take less time to prep. If you're grocery shopping on the same day as your prep, then you'll want to take the time for doing that into consideration too. I like to prep first thing in the morning (the earlier, the better); this way, I have the rest of the day free. No time is a bad time, just as long as you get it done. I recommend prepping the same day each week to build strong meal-prep habits. Sundays work best for most people, getting everything organized before the work week begins. Before you carve your prep day in stone, here are a couple of things to think about:

* **If you're crunched for time** or don't love eating foods you prepared on Sunday five or six days later, mini preps might work better for you. Mini preps are a great way to hammer out a few days' worth of food in a shorter amount of time. And if you're a frequent shopper (two to three times a week), it gives you a little more flexibility. Mini preps don't require you to pick up a week's worth of groceries all at once. From time to time, I'll do a mini prep on Sunday and again on Wednesday night to bring me into the weekend.

* **You may want to repeat some meals and snacks.** Most people say they want a varied meal plan, but when it comes down to it, easy trumps variety for most of us. Repeating a few meals and snacks will make your prep day simpler and greatly reduce your overall prep time. You can find sample plans to give you a head start on page 19.

Once you've decided on your recipes and locked down your prep day, you're ready to roll!

STEP ONE
GET CONTAINERS

In order to execute a smooth and organized meal prep, you must have the proper containers on hand. (Note: Once you have these containers, this step does not need to be repeated in your weekly meal-prep routine, except for the occasional purchase of resealable plastic bags.) There's nothing worse than not being able to find a suitable food container (or lid) for your beautifully planned and prepared meals. Having the right containers, organized and in reach, will not only speed up your prep and cleanup times, but will help you achieve your health goals too.

Chances are, you already have some containers at home. Are images of mismatched storage and take-out containers coming to mind? If you have a bunch of random containers in your kitchen, here's what you need to do:

1. Take out all your containers and lay them on a countertop or table.

2. Sort and set aside the ones with properly sealing lids.

3. From that pile, cross-reference the ones you have with the ones you still need (using the list below).

4. Make a list of containers you still need to complete the lineup.

5. Designate a specific spot in your kitchen for your weekly prep containers.

6. Donate or separately store extra containers.

If you don't have any suitable food-prep containers or need to supplement what you already have, use this list. Here are the exact amounts and sizes of containers to get you through an entire week:

* 8 glass containers: 1 quart (32 ounces, or 946 ml)

* 8 plastic containers: 1 quart (32 ounces, or 946 ml)

* 4 or 5 glass and/or plastic containers: 1 cup (8 ounces, or 240 ml)

* 4 or 5 glass and/or plastic containers: 1½ to 2 ounces (45 to 60 ml)

* 4 or 5 glass and/or plastic containers: 3 to 5 ounces (90 to 150 ml)

* 4 or 5 Mason jars: ½ pint (8 ounces, or 240 ml)

* 4 or 5 Mason jars: 1 quart (32 ounces, or 946 ml)

* Resealable plastic bags: sandwich size and snack size

* Plastic freezer bags: large/1 gallon (128 ounces, or 3.8 L)

Whether you're looking to lose weight, build muscle, or maintain your weight, you should prioritize using containers with appropriate portion sizes. Portion sizing is one of those elusive concepts that people think they have a good grasp on; however, most people underestimate the amount of food they eat in a sitting. (Note: Some people like food storage containers with dividers, but they aren't necessary.)

GLASS VS. PLASTIC CONTAINERS

I suggest having a mix of glass and plastic containers, as they serve different purposes.

Glass containers should be used for hot foods. They're safe for reheating meals in the microwave. If you eat right out of the container instead of transferring your meal to a plate, you'll only have one dish to wash—bonus! Speaking of washing, glass containers are super easy to clean and don't retain food odors and stains as much as plastic does.

Plastic containers should be reserved for cold food. They are affordable, portable, and suitable for meals that don't need to be heated. I love plastic containers—make sure they are BPA-free—because they stack neatly and take up less space. (Note: Plastic labelled "BPA-free" can still have chemicals that can leach out into your food. "Microwave-safe" labels often refer to how the plastic will hold up—it won't melt or crack—when heated in the microwave.)

STEP TWO
GROCERY SHOP

Grocery shopping is the catalyst of a successful food-prep session. Without a proper "grocery haul," there would be no prep. You may have seen #groceryhaul photos sweeping social media; it's a growing trend. These images detail the results of grocery-shopping expeditions, including filled shopping carts or food items sprawled out on countertops and tables. I love seeing these hauls. A healthy grocery haul leads to a healthy diet, right? Well, unfortunately, it's not that simple. Although your intention is to fill your cart with healthy foods, if you don't have a plan for all that goodness, some of those foods are likely to go to waste—we're all guilty of letting those veggies sit in the crisper to wilt and die; on the other hand, you may not have enough food to get you through the days you need it to. Whether you love or loathe grocery shopping, I want to call your attention to a few things and challenge you to reflect on your grocery-shopping habits. Can you make a few changes that will result in some healthier outcomes? Always!

SHOP ON A FULL STOMACH

Grocery shopping on an empty stomach presents a challenge—everything looks good! When you're hungry, bags of munchies and sweets can slip into the cart so fast, you won't even remember putting them there. I'm all about setting the stage for success, so let's make it a "rule" to have a snack or meal before heading out to the supermarket. I promise it will make it a lot easier to stick to your list, which brings me to the next tip . . .

MAKE AND BRING A LIST

It may seem obvious to go shopping with a list, but I want to emphasize how important this is for food-prep success. We've all gone to the grocery store and filled our carts with tons of food, only to get home and realize we can't make one decent meal out of what we have. The key is to stick to the list! To create a weekly list as an expert meal prepper, you need to include all the food items— fresh, frozen, boxed, and canned—to prepare your meals and snacks for the next five to seven days. Once you've picked the meals you want for the week, go through the recipes' lists of ingredients and add the items you don't already have in your kitchen to your list. Don't forget to take into account the number of people you'll be preparing meals for.

FOOD SHOPPING TERMS TO KNOW

Locally grown: This term refers to food, most often fruits and vegetables, that is grown near where you are located. Buying locally grown produce often means foods are fresher and pesticide-free. A farmers' market is the best place to find locally grown produce. Plus, buying directly from family farmers helps them stay in business.

Organic: Organic produce carries significantly less pesticide residue than conventional produce. Because organic regulations ban or severely restrict the use of food additives, this may be something for you to consider when buying fruits and vegetables in big-box grocery stores.

Whole foods: This term refers to foods that are unprocessed and unrefined, or processed and refined as little as possible. Whole foods typically do not contain added salt, sugars, or fat.

DON'T GET DISTRACTED

This is a helpful tip for any food shopper, not just preppers. Don't get distracted by food packaging with buzzwords like "fat-free" and "gluten-free"; they don't automatically make these foods healthy. There's a term for this distraction: health halo. It's given to foods that are perceived to be healthy, solely because of these claims. The problem with choosing foods based on the message on the package is that people tend to overbuy and overeat these foods. Stay out of the health-halo trap by following the next tip.

READ NUTRITION FACTS LABELS AND INGREDIENT LISTS

Foods without Nutrition Facts labels (fresh fruits and vegetables) are obvious healthy choices, but the reality is, foods in boxes, bags, and cans are abundant in our kitchens. So, it's your job to be a bit of a sleuth when buying these things, and reading packaging labels will tell you everything you need to know about what's inside. The great part is that once you've done this a few times, you'll establish your go-to food items and brands.

Deciphering the list of ingredients may seem like a big job, but I'm here to make it simple—I only want you to remember these two things:

* **Focus on the first two or three ingredients listed.** If you're seeing wholesome ingredients that you would use in a healthy recipe, you're on the right track. For example, if you're shopping for a healthy, whole grain variety of pasta, bread, or crackers, the word "whole" should appear as the first or second ingredient on the package (e.g., whole wheat, whole grain millet, whole grain brown rice flour). The ingredients used in the greatest amounts are listed first, followed by the ingredients with the smaller quantities in descending order.

* **The shorter the ingredient list, the better.** Some people even stick to the five-and-under rule. It definitely makes it easier to say yay or nay to a packaged food.

Manufacturers can be sneaky and try to "hide" sugar in the ingredient list by using a different source to add sweetness. Be aware that added sugar comes in many forms (over 50 forms to my knowledge). Here are a few common names to look out for: corn syrup, dextrin, honey, brown sugar, molasses, maple syrup, sucrose, dextrose, fructose, maltose, glucose rice syrup, cane syrup, coconut sugar, and beet sugar. It's best to avoid foods that have sugar in the top five ingredients or at all.

UNPACK AND ORGANIZE YOUR GROCERIES

Unpacking your groceries in an orderly fashion will put you a step closer to food-prep success. If you are prepping your meals as soon as you get home, the meats and other food items can be left on the counter for 10 to 15 minutes. If you need a little more time before cooking or are doing your prep the next day, place your perishable items in the refrigerator until you are ready to use them. I do suggest that you follow the next step, Clean and Cut, for produce before storing it in the refrigerator. As you empty your shopping bags, organize your items in the following way:

* Take fruits and vegetables out of their bags/packages and place them near the sink to be washed.

* Gather together the grains you'll be using for prep (rice, bread, pasta, quinoa, etc.) and leave them out on the counter; the rest can be put away.

* Group the meats (kept in their packaging).

STEP THREE
CLEAN AND CUT

This next section outlines the steps you need for a smooth meal-prep session. Washing and cutting produce in advance will keep you ahead of the game when it comes to preparing meals and healthy grab-and-go snacks, as well as save you time and money and eliminate food waste.

CLEAN

Before cleaning your produce, you want to start with a clean and sanitized prep area. Thoroughly wash your hands, counters and/or tables, chopping boards, and knives to avoid foodborne illnesses. To wash surfaces, simply use hot soapy water or an equal mixture of water and vinegar. Now that your space is ready, wash your fruits and vegetables to reduce your exposure to pesticides and bacteria and to extend the life of your produce. You can leave the fruits and vegetables whole or cut them into smaller pieces before washing them.

To wash your produce, fill a clean sink with fresh, cool water (or a plastic tub with 8 cups, or 2 L, of water) and add ½ lemon (juice and rind) and ¼ cup (60 ml) of vinegar. Place your fruits and vegetables in the sink. Let the produce sit for 10 minutes. During this time, take out additional items you'll need for prepping (e.g., peelers, knives, bowls, salad spinner, etc.). After 10 minutes, agitate the fruits and vegetables, let the water out, and give them a quick rinse under cool water before placing them on a clean dish towel to dry. (Note: For delicate fruits, such as berries, separately wash them in a smaller bowl or container and let them sit for a shorter amount of time.)

CUT

Divide your vegetables into two categories: to be **cooked** and to be kept raw. Vegetables to be cooked may include zucchini, bell peppers, broccoli, asparagus, potatoes, etc. Cut these vegetables according to the recipe you are following (e.g., large pieces, roughly the same size, for roasting and stir-frying or diced for sautéing). Once cut, toss them into the pan, skillet, oven dish or baking sheet they will be cooked in. Vegetables to keep **raw** may include celery, carrots, snap peas, bell peppers, cherry tomatoes, etc. Either slice the vegetables lengthwise for snacking and/or dice them for adding to meals according to the recipes you have chosen (e.g., salads and wraps). Once the vegetables are cut, place them in appropriate-size containers to store in the refrigerator or leave out on a large plate until you're ready to add them to your dishes.

PRO PREP TIP

If you are not prepping immediately, keep your cleaned fruits and vegetables fresh by drying them with a paper towel or clean dishcloth before storing them in an airtight container and placing them in the refrigerator's crisper or temperature-controlled drawer.

COOK

This step is when ultimate time-saving and efficiency comes into play. Having two or three items cooking at once will greatly speed up the prepping process. Using the stovetop and oven at the same time is the best way to get your prep done. If you're new to cooking in this way or new to prepping, this multitasking will become second nature—it just takes a little practice. These are general guidelines for cooking multiple recipes. The advantage of using the recipes in this book is that they don't have super-long cooking or marinating times.

Remember, you don't have to prep an entire week's worth of food on your first go. Use these instructions to nail your prep even if you're only cooking two dishes. You will be able to add more recipes each week to build up to the number of meals you would ideally like to have done on your prep day. For examples of how to apply this step, see the cooking instructions for the meal plans in the Five Meal-Prep Plans to Get You Started section starting on page 19.

SCAN THE RECIPES FOR INGREDIENTS THAT WILL TAKE LONGEST TO COOK
Once those items (e.g., roasting vegetables) are cooking, prepare the next part of these recipes (e.g., sauces). Then move on to the ingredients with the second-longest cooking times (e.g., meat, grains), and so on. When you have a few items baking and simmering, you will have time to prep the no-cook recipes; for example, you can start assembling salads or overnight oats into jars.

PREHEAT THE OVEN
Preheating will result in even cooking, so as soon as you come across the words "preheat the oven" in a recipe, turn it on. Most foods have flexible cooking temperatures, so if a recipe instructs you to cook something at 400°F (200°C) and something else at 450°F (230°C), it's completely acceptable to set your oven temperature in the middle at 425°F (220°C). Please note, this does not apply to baking, where the cooking temperatures are more exact.

SWITCH RACK POSITIONS OF PANS HALFWAY THROUGH COOKING TIME
Doing this is especially necessary for even cooking if you have two or more items in the oven and are using both racks. Let's say a recipe specifies to use a particular rack: simply swap the position of the dishes from top to bottom and vice versa halfway through cooking. You should also swap racks and rotate dishes if you feel the food is getting too brown in one area.

TEST FOR DONENESS
When you are cooking multiple items in the oven at the same time, different foods will most likely be done at varying times. Cooking times can also increase when cooking a few items at once, so keep an eye on things and promptly remove items from the oven when they're done.

PRO PREP TIP

If having a huge mound of dishes to wash has repelled you from cooking in big batches before, do your best to eliminate some dishes as you prep. Once something is cooked, start filling your containers up and wash the pan or pot as you go.

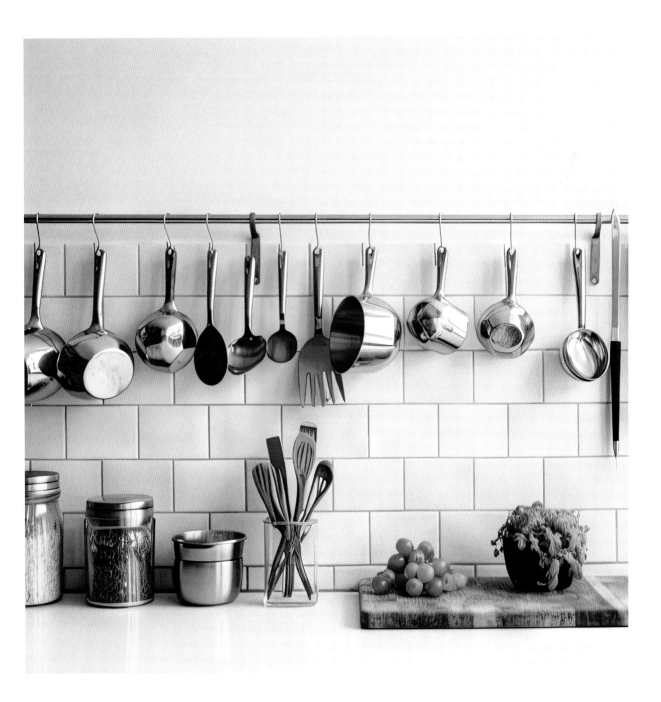

PORTION AND PACK

There are two methods for portioning and packing: batch, or bulk, and individual meals. The recipes you decide to prep for the week will determine which method you use. Think of **batch, or bulk, packing** as "buffet-style" meal prep, separately storing meats, vegetables, and grains. When it's time to eat, you take a portion from each container to make a complete meal (e.g., chicken, broccoli, and quinoa). **Packing individual meals** means portioning out the finished meal into containers so it is ready to go. Meals like stir-fries, stuffed potatoes, and overnight oats are good examples of this. You may want to try both methods in the beginning to see which one works best for you. And before placing containers in the refrigerator, make sure any cooked foods have completely cooled to avoid increasing the fridge temperature.

BATCH PACKING

Pros

* More flexibility when putting meals together.

* Can switch up food pairings and add different seasonings when serving/eating.

* Works well when feeding people with different food preferences.

Cons

* Need additional large containers to store foods separately.

* More dishes to wash.

INDIVIDUAL MEALS

Pros

* Grab and go.

* Can eat your meal straight from the packed container.

* Fewer dishes to wash.

Cons

* Less flexibility when putting meals together.

approved food list

ANIMAL-BASED (Protein)

chicken breast
eggs
lean ground beef
lean ground chicken
salmon (wild)
shrimp
sirloin steak
tilapia
tuna (fresh and canned, packed in water)
turkey breast

PLANT-BASED (Protein)

black beans
chia seeds
chickpeas
edamame
lentils
peanuts
quinoa
seitan
tempeh
tofu

DAIRY (Protein and Some Healthy Fat)

cheese (cheddar, feta, mozzarella, Parmesan, ricotta)
cottage cheese
Greek yogurt
skim milk

GRAINS (Carbohydrate)

barley
brown rice
oats
popcorn
quinoa
soba noodles
spelt pasta
whole grain bread
whole grain pasta
whole wheat tortillas

VEGETABLES (Carbohydrate)

alfalfa sprouts
asparagus
avocados
beets
bok choy
broccoli
brussels sprouts
cabbage
carrots
cauliflower
celery
corn (canned)
cucumbers
garlic
green beans
kale
lettuce (romaine)
mushrooms
olives
onions
parsley
peas
peppers
spinach
squash
tomatoes (fresh and canned)
zucchini

FRUITS (Carbohydrate)

apples
bananas
blackberries
blueberries
cantaloupe
cherries
coconut
grapefruit
kiwi
lemons
limes
mangos
melon
nectarines
oranges
papaya
peaches
pears
pineapples
raspberries
strawberries
watermelon

BEANS (Carbohydrate and Protein)

black beans
chickpeas
edamame
kidney beans
lentils
white (cannellini) beans

NUTS AND SEEDS (Healthy Fat and Protein)

almonds
chia seeds
flax seeds
peanuts
pumpkin seeds
sesame seeds
sunflower seeds
walnuts

OILS/VINEGARS

avocado oil
balsamic vinegar
coconut oil
extra-virgin olive oil
red wine vinegar

SEASONINGS

almond extract
basil
cayenne pepper
cinnamon
cumin
curry powder
garlic powder
ginger (ground)
Himalayan pink salt
nutmeg
onion powder
oregano
parsley
rosemary
sage
thyme
turmeric
vanilla extract

NATURAL SWEETENERS

coconut palm sugar
honey (raw and unfiltered)
maple syrup (pure)
stevia

BEVERAGES

almond milk (unsweetened)
coconut milk (unsweetened)
coffee
herbal tea
soy milk (unsweetened)

CONDIMENTS AND PREPARED SAUCES

broth (chicken and vegetable, low sodium)
hot sauce
mustard
salsa
soy sauce (low sodium)
tomato paste

WHAT ARE MACRONUTRIENTS?

Macronutrients, often referred to as "macros," are the three basic components of every diet: proteins, carbohydrates, and essential fatty acids (or healthy fats). Although many foods fall into more than one macro category, one usually serves as the primary source. Here's a quick look at how each of the macros are used in the body:

Proteins are the main component of muscles, organs, and glands. Your best sources of protein are found in meat, dairy, and nuts.

Carbohydrates have one main function, which is to provide energy for the body, especially the brain and the nervous system. Whole grain bread and pasta, oats, legumes, and starchy vegetables are all good complex carbohydrate sources.

Essential fatty acids play a part in many metabolic processes, and there is evidence to suggest that low levels of essential fatty acids, or the wrong balance of types among them, may be a factor in a number of illnesses. Fish and shellfish, flaxseed, olive oil, pumpkin seeds, sunflower seeds, nuts, and avocados are examples of healthy fats.

five meal-prep plans to get you started

HIGH-PROTEIN PLAN

BREAKFAST
Breakfast Burritos 36
Cheesy Egg Bites 38

MAINS
Roasted Vegetables and Chicken Wraps (made
    with the three-ingredient wraps in the Pro
    Prep Tip) 76
Ground Chicken and Quinoa–Stuffed Peppers 79
Mixed Bean Salad 89
Mediterranean Chicken with Crispy Sweet Potato
    Medallions 80 and 125

SNACKS
Chia Seed Pudding 43
High-Protein Chocolate Chip Banana Bread 107
Very Berry Smoothie 50
Fruit Dip Delight with Sliced Fruit (apples,
    strawberries, bananas, cantaloupe) 138

	BREAKFAST	SNACK	LUNCH	SNACK	DINNER
Day 1	Breakfast Burritos	Chia Seed Pudding	Roasted Vegetables and Chicken Wraps	High-Protein Chocolate Chip Banana Bread	Ground Chicken and Quinoa–Stuffed Peppers
Day 2	Breakfast Burritos	Very Berry Smoothie	Roasted Vegetables and Chicken Wraps	Fruit Dip Delight with Sliced Fruit	Ground Chicken and Quinoa–Stuffed Peppers
Day 3	Cheesy Egg Bites	Chia Seed Pudding	Mixed Bean Salad	High-Protein Chocolate Chip Banana Bread	Mediterranean Chicken with Crispy Sweet Potato Medallions
Day 4	Cheesy Egg Bites	Very Berry Smoothie	Mixed Bean Salad	Fruit Dip Delight with Sliced Fruit	Mediterranean Chicken with Crispy Sweet Potato Medallions

HIGH-PROTEIN PLAN: COOKING INSTRUCTIONS

Before you start prepping this meal plan, take a moment to ask yourself these two questions: Are you prepping for the entire four days in one meal-prep session or are you doing two mini preps? And are you prepping for one or two people? If you're planning two mini preps, decide which meals you would like to prep during each session. This could mean breakfast and lunches in one session and dinner and snacks in another, or any combination that works best for you. And if you're only prepping for one person, you will need to cut the recipes in half. Here are the steps for prepping the entire four days in one session:

1. Get out all the containers that are required so you can assemble and pack your meals as each food item is prepared.

2. Preheat the oven to 350°F (190°C) for the High-Protein Chocolate Chip Banana Bread. Follow the recipe for the High-Protein Chocolate Chip Banana Bread. Bake in the preheated oven.

3. Meanwhile, wash and cut the vegetables for the Breakfast Burritos, Cheesy Egg Bites, Roasted Vegetables and Chicken Wraps, Crispy Sweet Potato Medallions, and Mediterranean Chicken. Leave the bell peppers whole for the Ground Chicken and Quinoa–Stuffed Peppers. Also dice the vegetables for the Mixed Bean Salad, drain and rinse the beans, and follow the instructions for the dressing. Assemble the salad and store it in the refrigerator.

4. In a large skillet, prepare the chicken for the Mediterranean Chicken and Chicken Wraps in the same pan. Once cooked, remove the portion needed for the wraps, then continue with the steps for the Mediterranean Chicken.

5. When cooked completely, remove the baked Chocolate Chip Banana Bread from the oven. Increase the oven temperature to 375°F (190°C) and cook the vegetables for the Roasted Vegetable and Chicken Wraps.

6. Place the finished Mediterranean Chicken in containers. Rinse the skillet and cook the eggs for the Breakfast Burritos. At the same time, prepare a separate skillet and cook the Crispy Sweet Potato Medallions.

7. Once the vegetables are roasted, remove from the oven, add to the wraps, and assemble. Leave the oven on at 375°F (190°C). Add the cooked eggs to tortillas, assemble the Breakfast Burritos, and place them in the oven. While they cook, follow the instructions for cooking the Cheesy Egg Cups, adding them to the oven once prepared. Remove both egg dishes when finished according to their cook times.

8. Once the potatoes are done, cook the filling for the Ground Chicken and Quinoa Stuffed–Peppers. Once the filling is done, add it to the bell peppers and cook according to the recipe.

9. While the Stuffed Peppers cook, prepare the Chia Seed Pudding.

Note: The Fruit Dip Delight with Sliced Fruit and Very Berry Smoothie can be quickly made the day you are going to eat them.

GLUTEN-FREE PLAN

BREAKFAST
Easy Egg Scramble with a Piece of Fruit 34
Healthy Booster Smoothie with a Small Handful
    of Almonds 49

MAINS
Thai Bowls with Peanut Sauce 66
Colorful Fish Tacos 73
Classic and Lean Chili 74
Pesto Tilapia with Crispy Sweet Potato
    Medallions 67 and 125

SNACKS
Roasted Chickpeas 129
Tropical Energy Balls 105
Superfood Popcorn 121
Vegetables with Greek Yogurt Dip 119

	BREAKFAST	SNACK	LUNCH	SNACK	DINNER
Day 1	Healthy Booster Smoothie with a Small Handful of Almonds	Roasted Chickpeas	Thai Bowls with Peanut Sauce	Tropical Energy Balls	Classic and Lean Chili
Day 2	Healthy Booster Smoothie with a Small Handful of Almonds	Roasted Chickpeas	Thai Bowls with Peanut Sauce	Superfood Popcorn	Pesto Tilapia with Crispy Sweet Potato Medallions
Day 3	Easy Egg Scramble with a Piece of Fruit	Vegetables with Greek Yogurt Dip	Colorful Fish Tacos	Tropical Energy Balls	Classic and Lean Chili
Day 4	Easy Egg Scramble with a Piece of Fruit	Vegetables with Greek Yogurt Dip	Colorful Fish Tacos	Superfood Popcorn	Pesto Tilapia with Crispy Sweet Potato Medallions

GLUTEN-FREE PLAN: COOKING INSTRUCTIONS

Before you start prepping this meal plan, take a moment to ask yourself these two questions: Are you prepping for the entire four days in one meal-prep session or are you doing two mini preps? And are you prepping for one or two people? If you're planning two mini preps, decide which meals you would like to prep during each session. This could mean breakfast and lunches in one session and dinner and snacks in another, or any combination that works best for you. And if you're only prepping for one person, you will need to cut the recipes in half. Here are the steps for prepping the entire four days in one session:

1. Get out all the containers that are required so you can assemble and pack your meals as each food item is prepared.

2. Preheat the oven to 400°F (200°C) for the Roasted Chickpeas. Marinate the fish for the Colorful Fish Tacos and make the pesto for the Pesto Tilapia, if not using store-bought pesto. Place the chickpeas in the preheated oven.

3. Using the stovetop, cook the Crispy Sweet Potato Medallions and make the brown rice for the Thai Bowls with Peanut Sauce according to package directions. Once these are done, place them into containers and let cool.

4. While the sweet potatoes and rice cook, make the Tropical Energy Balls and Superfood Popcorn, and pack into containers. Immediately refrigerate the Tropical Energy Balls.

5. Remove the chickpeas from the oven, reduce the oven heat to 375°F (190°C), and place the marinated fish for the Colorful Fish Tacos in the oven. Place the Roasted Chickpeas into containers and let cool.

6. Moving back to the stovetop, start making the Classic and Lean Chili, the Easy Egg Scramble, and the fish for the Pesto Tilapia at the same time. Start with the chili, and once the ground meat is browning, tend to the Easy Egg Scramble and the tilapia.

7. Remove the fish for the Colorful Fish Tacos from the oven and place into containers to cool. Finish cooking the Easy Egg Scramble and the fish for the Pesto Tilapia and place into containers to cool (place the fish for the Pesto Tilapia into the containers with the Crispy Sweet Potato Medallions). Continue cooking the chili recipe.

8. In the meantime, make, pack, and refrigerate the Greek Yogurt Dip, the Avocado Aioli for the Colorful Fish Tacos, and the peanut sauce for the Thai Bowls with Peanut Sauce. Also pack and refrigerate the vegetables for the Vegetables with Greek Yogurt Dip and the toppings for the Colorful Fish Tacos.

9. Assemble, pack, and refrigerate the Thai Bowls with Peanut Sauce.

10. Lastly, place the Classic and Lean Chili into containers and let cool before refrigerating.

DAIRY-FREE PLAN

BREAKFAST
Chocolate Raspberry Breakfast Quinoa 51
Pineapple-Ginger Green Smoothie and Whole
  Wheat Bread with Almond Butter 50

MAINS
"Not Your Mama's Meatloaf" Muffins 93
Ginger-Soy Chicken Thighs 82
Tomato, Egg, and Lentil Bowls 84
Chicken and Bacon Club Wraps 58

SNACKS
Pumpkin-Spice Granola with Coconut Milk
  Yogurt 114
Sweet-and-Salty Trail Mix 115
Healthier Tuna Salad with Super Seed
  Crackers 116
Energy-Bite Cookies 111

	BREAKFAST	SNACK	LUNCH	SNACK	DINNER
Day 1	Pineapple-Ginger Green Smoothie and Whole Wheat Bread with Almond Butter	Healthier Tuna Salad with Super Seed Crackers	Tomato, Egg, and Lentil Bowls	Pumpkin-Spice Granola with Coconut Milk Yogurt	"Not Your Mama's Meatloaf" Muffins
Day 2	Pineapple-Ginger Green Smoothie and Whole Wheat Bread with Almond Butter	Energy-Bite Cookies	Tomato, Egg, and Lentil Bowls	Sweet-and-Salty Trail Mix	Ginger-Soy Chicken Thighs
Day 3	Chocolate Raspberry Breakfast Quinoa	Healthier Tuna Salad with Super Seed Crackers	Chicken and Bacon Club Wraps	Pumpkin-Spice Granola with Coconut Milk Yogurt	"Not Your Mama's Meatloaf" Muffins
Day 4	Chocolate Raspberry Breakfast Quinoa	Energy-Bite Cookies	Chicken and Bacon Club Wraps	Sweet-and-Salty Trail Mix	Ginger-Soy Chicken Thighs

DAIRY-FREE PLAN: COOKING INSTRUCTIONS

Before you start prepping this meal plan, take a moment to ask yourself these two questions: Are you prepping for the entire four days in one meal-prep session or are you doing two mini preps? And are you prepping for one or two people? If you're planning two mini preps, decide which meals you would like to prep during each session. This could mean breakfast and lunches in one session and dinner and snacks in another, or any combination that works best for you. And if you're only prepping for one person, you will need to cut the recipes in half. Here are the steps for prepping the entire four days in one session:

1. Get out all the containers that are required so you can assemble and pack your meals as each food item is prepared.

2. Preheat the oven to 375°F (190°C) for the "Not Your Mama's Meatloaf" Muffins and Ginger-Soy Chicken Thighs. Make the meatloaf muffins and marinate the chicken thighs. Place both dishes into the oven.

3. On the stovetop, make the Chocolate Raspberry Breakfast Quinoa and use the traditional stovetop method for cooking hard-boiled eggs for the Tomato, Egg, and Lentil Bowls. (Set the eggs in a pot of cold water and bring to a boil with the lid on. Once the water boils, turn off the heat and let the eggs sit, covered, for 15 minutes or so before running under cold water.)

4. In the meantime, make the Sweet-and-Salty Trail Mix, the Pumpkin-Spice Granola, and the Energy-Bite Cookies. Place the trail mix into containers and set aside the granola and cookies to bake later.

5. When the quinoa and hard-boiled eggs are done on the stovetop, place the quinoa into containers and let cool and peel and slice the hard-boiled eggs.

6. Using the stovetop, cook the chicken and bacon for the Chicken and Bacon Club Wraps.

7. Remove the meatloaf muffins and chicken thighs, place into containers, and let cool. Reduce the oven heat to 325°F (170°C) and place the Pumpkin-Spice Granola and Energy-Bite Cookies into the oven.

8. In the meantime, assemble the Tomato, Egg, and Lentil Bowls; assemble the Chicken and Bacon Club Wraps; make the Healthier Tuna Salad; and prep the ingredients for the Pineapple-Ginger Green Smoothies in advance (if you want; or you can quickly make the same day you're going to drink it).

9. Remove the granola and cookies from the oven, place into containers, and let cool.

10. Lastly, refrigerate everything, once cooled, except the Sweet-and-Salty Trail Mix.

VEGETARIAN PLAN

BREAKFAST
Berry Vanilla High-Protein Pancakes 46
Mocha Monkey Smoothie 49

MAINS
Ultimate Black Bean Burgers 56
Falafel Bowls 70
Superfood Green Salad 63
Vegetable and Tofu Skewers 68

SNACKS
Apple Cinnamon Walnut Muffins 108
Peanut Butter Brownies 103
Chocolate Granola with Greek Yogurt 113
Nut Butter Roll-Ups 121

	BREAKFAST	SNACK	LUNCH	SNACK	DINNER
Day 1	Berry Vanilla High-Protein Pancakes	Nut Butter Roll-Ups	Superfood Green Salad	Chocolate Granola with Greek Yogurt	Ultimate Black Bean Burgers
Day 2	Berry Vanilla High-Protein Pancakes	Nut Butter Roll-Ups	Superfood Green Salad	Chocolate Granola with Greek Yogurt	Ultimate Black Bean Burgers
Day 3	Mocha Monkey Smoothie	Apple Cinnamon Walnut Muffins	Falafel Bowls	Peanut Butter Brownies	Vegetable and Tofu Skewers
Day 4	Mocha Monkey Smoothie	Apple Cinnamon Walnut Muffins	Falafel Bowls	Peanut Butter Brownies	Vegetable and Tofu Skewers

VEGETARIAN PLAN: COOKING INSTRUCTIONS

Before you start prepping this meal plan, take a moment to ask yourself these two questions: Are you prepping for the entire four days in one meal-prep session or are you doing two mini preps? And are you prepping for one or two people? If you're planning two mini preps, decide which meals you would like to prep during each session. This could mean breakfast and lunches in one session and dinner and snacks in another, or any combination that works best for you. And if you're only prepping for one person, you will need to cut the recipes in half. Here are the steps for prepping the entire four days in one session:

1. The night before prep day, soak the dried chickpeas overnight for the falafel in the Falafel Bowls.

2. On prep day, get out all the containers that are required so you can assemble and pack your meals as each food item is prepared.

3. Make the falafel dough for the Falafel Bowls and refrigerate the dough for about an hour before cooking.

4. Preheat the oven to 350°F (180°C). Make the batter for the Apple Cinnamon Walnut Muffins and mix together the Chocolate Granola. Place both in the preheated oven.

5. On the stovetop, cook the quinoa for the Superfood Green Salad according to package directions.

6. In the meantime, rinse and drain the black beans for the Ultimate Black Bean Burgers, remove the excess liquid from the tofu for the Vegetable and Tofu Skewers, and assemble the Superfood Green Salad and the bowls of the Falafel Bowls directly in the containers. Refrigerate the Falafel Bowls containers.

7. Remove the Chocolate Granola from the oven and let cool. Make the Ultimate Black Bean Burgers, shape the falafel dough for the Falafel Bowls, and assemble the skewers for the Vegetable and Tofu skewers. Cook the burgers and falafel in separate skillets on the stovetop.

8. Remove the muffins from the oven and let cool, along with the cooked burgers and falafel. Increase the oven heat to broil and cook the Vegetable and Tofu Skewers.

9. Make the salad dressing for the Superfood Green Salad, pack it into containers, and place in the refrigerator. Prep the ingredients for the Mocha Monkey Smoothies in advance (if you want; or you can quickly make the same day you're going to drink it).

10. Add the quinoa to the containers with the assembled Superfood Green Salad and refrigerate. Pack and refrigerate the falafel, burgers (with any toppings in separate containers), skewers, muffins, and granola.

11. Lastly, make, pack, and refrigerate the Berry Vanilla High-Protein Pancakes and the Peanut Butter Brownies.

Note: The Nut Butter Roll-Ups can be quickly made the day you are going to eat them.

LOW-CARB PLAN

BREAKFAST

Egg and Cheese English Muffin Sandwiches 41

Feta, Tomato, and Spinach Omelet 33

MAINS

Zucchini Noodles Caprese-Style with Sliced
   Chicken 61

Mediterranean Steak Salad with a Piece of
   Fruit 65

Pan-Fried Teriyaki Salmon with Cauliflower
   Rice 87 and 124

Steak Fajitas (low-carb option in recipe) 98

SNACKS

Sweet-and-Salty Trail Mix with Greek Yogurt 115

Amazeballs 110

Vegetable Sticks with Hummus 136

Baked Tortilla Triangles with Salsa and Avocado
   Aioli 128, 134, and 135

	BREAKFAST	SNACK	LUNCH	SNACK	DINNER
Day 1	Egg and Cheese English Muffin Sandwiches	Sweet-and-Salty Trail Mix with Greek Yogurt	Mediterranean Steak Salad with a Piece of Fruit	Amazeballs	Pan-Fried Teriyaki Salmon with Cauliflower Rice
Day 2	Egg and Cheese English Muffin Sandwiches	Vegetable Sticks with Hummus	Mediterranean Steak Salad with a Piece of Fruit	Amazeballs	Pan-Fried Teriyaki Salmon with Cauliflower Rice
Day 3	Feta, Tomato, and Spinach Omelet	Sweet-and-Salty Trail Mix with Greek Yogurt	Zucchini Noodles Caprese-Style with Sliced Chicken	Baked Tortilla Triangles with Salsa and Avocado Aioli	Steak Fajitas (low-carb option in recipe)
Day 4	Feta, Tomato, and Spinach Omelet	Vegetable Sticks with Hummus	Zucchini Noodles Caprese-Style with Sliced Chicken	Baked Tortilla Triangles with Salsa and Avocado Aioli	Steak Fajitas (low-carb option in recipe)

LOW-CARB PLAN: COOKING INSTRUCTIONS

Before you start prepping this meal plan, take a moment to ask yourself these two questions: Are you prepping for the entire four days in one meal-prep session or are you doing two mini preps? And are you prepping for one or two people? If you're planning two mini preps, decide which meals you would like to prep during each session. This could mean breakfast and lunches in one session and dinner and snacks in another, or any combination that works best for you. And if you're only prepping for one person, you will need to cut the recipes in half. Here are the steps for prepping the entire four days in one session:

1. Get out all the containers that are required so you can assemble and pack your meals as each food item is prepared.

2. Start cooking the proteins, as they typically take longer to prepare. Use 2 skillets, 1 for the chicken in the Zucchini Noodles Caprese-Style (follow the directions for cooking chicken in the Chicken and Bacon Club Wrap on page 58) and 1 for the steak in the Mediterranean Steak Salad. Marinate the steak, bell peppers, and onion for the Steak Fajitas recipes.

3. Meanwhile, make the Feta, Tomato, and Spinach Omelet. Slice the steak, chicken, and omelet and place into separate containers. Rinse both skillets to use in step 6.

4. Preheat the oven to 350°F (180°C). Assemble the salad for the Mediterranean Steak Salad directly in the containers and pack the vegetable sticks for the Hummus. Place the eggs for the Egg and Cheese English Muffin Sandwiches, the Sweet-and-Salty Trail Mix, and the Baked Tortilla Triangles into the preheated oven.

5. Meanwhile, cook the turkey bacon for the Egg and Cheese English Muffin Sandwiches. In a separate skillet, cook the salmon for the Pan-Fried Teriyaki Salmon. While these cook, spiralize the zucchini for the Zucchini Noodles Caprese-Style and process the cauliflower for the Cauliflower Rice. When the salmon is done, place into containers and use the same skillet to cook the riced cauliflower.

6. Remove the items from the oven as they finish cooking and set aside to cool. Increase the oven temperature to 425°F (220°C) to cook the fajita filling for the Steak Fajitas. While the fajita filling cooks, assemble and pack the Egg and Cheese English Muffin Sandwiches and the Zucchini Noodles Caprese-Style and add the Cauliflower Rice to salmon containers. Place the containers in the refrigerator.

7. Make the condiments: the salad dressing for the Mediterranean Steak Salad, the Hummus, the Salsa and Avocado Aioli for the Baked Tortilla Triangles, and the Guacamole (if using) and Spicy Greek Yogurt Dip (if using) for the Steak Fajitas.

8. Pack the Baked Tortilla Triangles, the Sweet-and-Salty Trail Mix, and the fajita filling for the Steak Fajitas, along with the condiments. Refrigerate everything but the Baked Tortilla Triangles.

9. Lastly, make, pack, and refrigerate the Amazeballs.

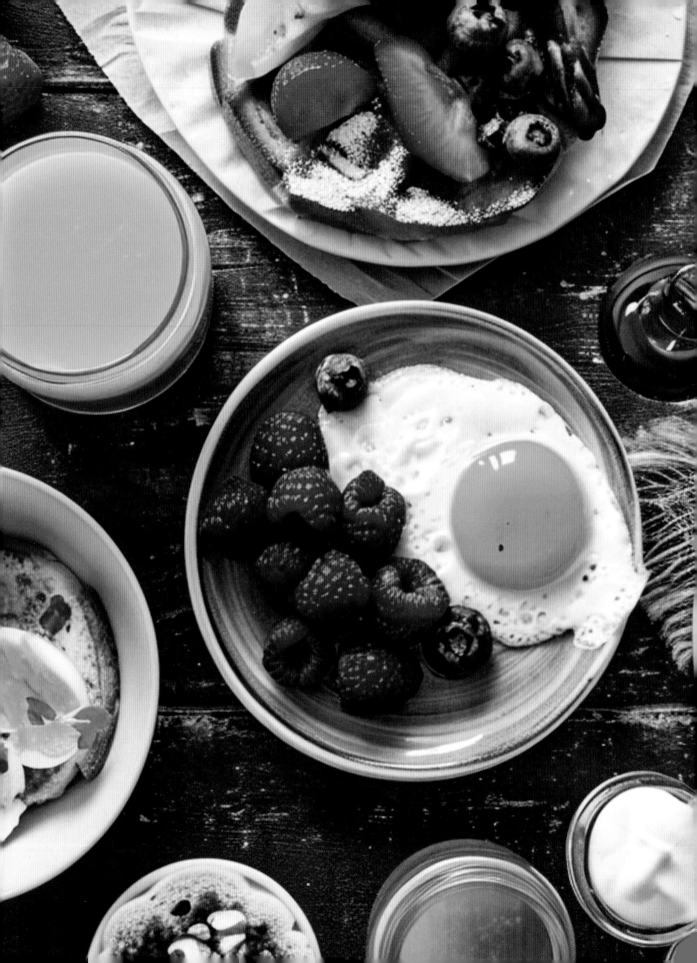

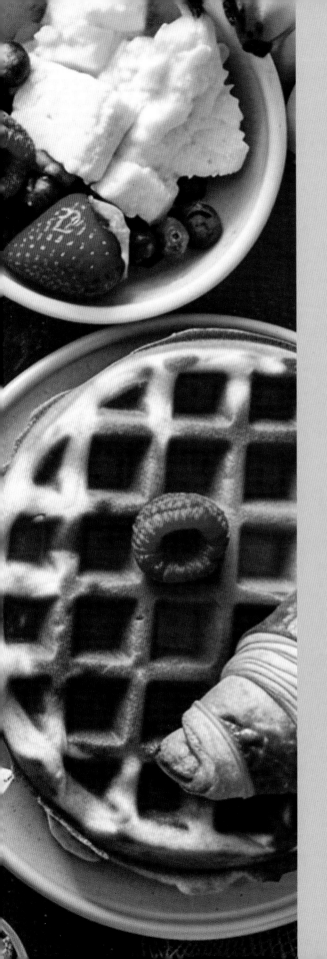

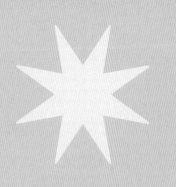

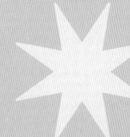

BREAKFAST

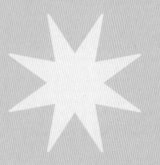

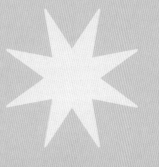

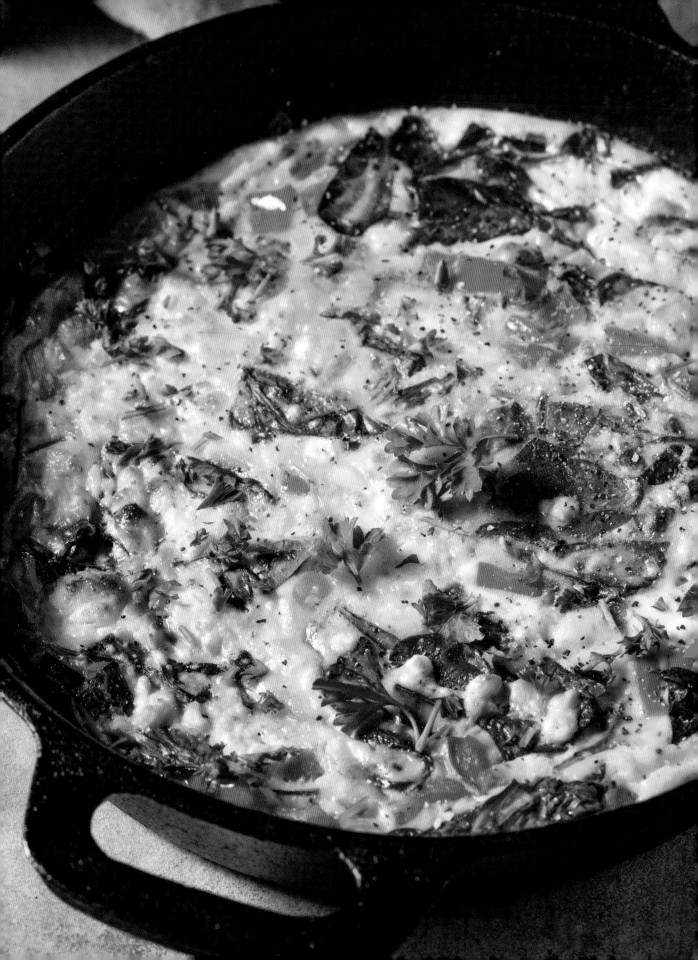

Feta, Tomato, and Spinach Omelet

Yield: 4 portions

Prep Time: 10 minutes

Cook Time: 10 minutes

Omelets for meal prep? You bet! Plus, you don't have to reserve them for breakfast. They're great for any meal of the day.

1 tablespoon (15 ml) extra-virgin olive oil

5 large eggs

2 egg whites

Himalayan pink salt, to taste

Freshly ground black pepper, to taste

¾ cup (23 g) chopped spinach

¼ cup (38 g) crumbled feta cheese

6 cherry tomatoes, halved

1. Heat the olive oil in a large skillet over medium heat for 30 seconds.

2. In a large bowl, whisk together the eggs and egg whites with the salt and black pepper.

3. Pour the egg mixture into the heated skillet and swirl until the eggs cover the entire bottom of the skillet. Cook for 1 to 2 minutes.

4. Arrange the spinach, feta, and tomatoes on one side of the egg mixture. Cook until the edges of the eggs begin to curl up, 2 to 3 minutes. Loosen the omelet from the skillet using a spatula and fold it in half over the filling. Continue cooking for 2 to 3 more minutes.

5. Transfer the omelet to a large plate or cutting board. Let the omelet sit for 1 to 2 minutes.

6. Slice into 4 pie slices and place each slice into a container. Store in the refrigerator for up to 5 days. To reheat, warm the omelet in a skillet over low heat for 3 to 5 minutes, turning once, until it is heated through or microwave for 50 to 60 seconds.

Easy Egg Scramble

This egg scramble is fantastic on its own, but if you are looking for an accompaniment for it, a couple slices of toasted rye bread, or my favorite, a whole wheat English muffin, can easily round out this meal.

Yield: 4 portions

Prep Time: 10 minutes

Cook Time: 10 minutes

2 teaspoons extra-virgin olive oil

¼ cup (18 g) chopped mushrooms

¼ cup (40 g) diced onion of your choice

¼ cup (35 g) diced red bell pepper

6 large eggs

¼ cup (60 ml) milk

¼ cup (45 g) chopped tomato

¼ cup (30 g) shredded cheddar cheese

1 cup (245 g) Salsa (page 134)

1. Heat the olive oil in a large skillet over medium heat for 30 seconds.

2. Add the mushrooms, onion, and bell pepper to the skillet, and cook and stir for 2 to 3 minutes.

3. While the vegetables are cooking, crack the eggs into a large bowl, add the milk, and whisk together until combined.

4. Add the egg mixture and the chopped tomato to the vegetables in the skillet. Cook for 4 to 5 minutes, stirring frequently to scramble all the ingredients together until the eggs are completely cooked through. Turn off the heat, sprinkle the shredded cheese on top of the egg scramble, and let the cheese melt slightly.

5. Equally divide the scramble into 4 containers, storing the salsa in separate small containers. Store in the refrigerator for up to 4 days. When ready to enjoy, microwave for 45 seconds and top with the salsa.

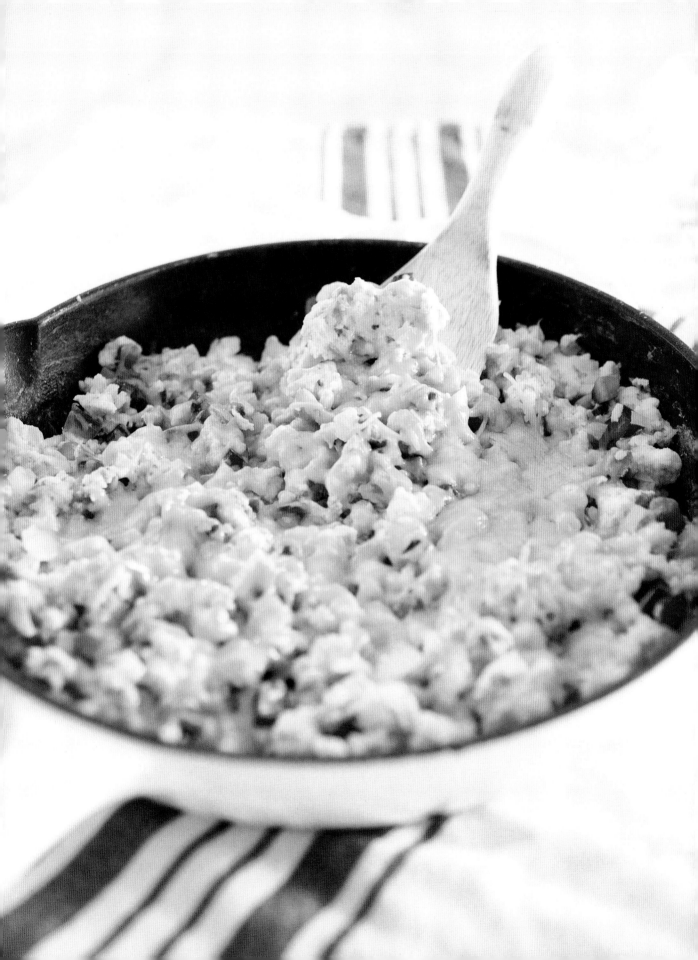

Breakfast Burritos

These breakfast burritos are great not only for meal prep, but also for serving a crowd.

Yield: 4 portions

Prep Time: 15 minutes

Cook Time: 10 minutes

5 large eggs

3 egg whites

¼ cup (60 g) canned black beans, rinsed and drained

¼ cup (40 g) diced red onion

⅓ cup (50 g) diced green bell pepper

½ cup (75 g) halved grape tomatoes

¼ cup (35 g) seeded and diced jalapeño (optional)

2 tablespoons (30 ml) cold water

¼ teaspoon cumin

¼ teaspoon chili powder

½ teaspoon Himalayan pink salt

1 tablespoon (15 ml) olive oil

4 large (10 inches, or 25 cm, each) whole wheat tortillas

¼ cup (30 g) shredded sharp cheddar cheese

1 cup (245 g) Salsa (page 134), for serving

¼ cup (30 g) Guacamole (page 133), for serving

1. Preheat the oven to 375°F (190°C). Line a large baking sheet with aluminum foil and set aside.

2. In a large bowl, whisk together the eggs and egg whites. Add the black beans, onion, bell pepper, tomatoes, jalapeño, cold water, cumin, chili powder, and pink salt, and mix together.

3. Heat the olive oil in a large skillet over medium-low heat for 30 seconds. Pour the egg mixture into the heated skillet and swirl until the eggs cover the entire bottom of the skillet. Cook until the edges of the eggs begin to curl up, 3 to 4 minutes. Loosen the omelet from the skillet using a spatula and fold it in half. Continue cooking until the eggs are set and cooked through, 2 to 3 minutes more. The omelet may be flipped once more if it gets too brown on one side.

4. Lay out the tortillas on a clean surface. Evenly divide the omelet among the tortillas, placing it on one-half of each tortilla. Sprinkle the cheese on top of each omelet. Wrap the tortillas around the omelet by tucking in the ends and rolling. Place the burritos, seam sides down, on the prepared baking sheet.

5. Bake for 5 to 6 minutes, until the burritos begin to turn golden brown. Carefully watch the burritos so they don't burn. Remove from the oven and let the burritos cool slightly. Diagonally slice the burritos in half and place into 4 containers. Divide the salsa and guacamole into small containers to serve with the burritos. Store in the refrigerator for up to 4 days. To reheat, place the burrito on a baking sheet and cook in the oven for about 15 minutes at 325°F (170°C) or microwave for 30 to 50 seconds. Serve with the salsa and guacamole.

Hard-Boiled Eggs in the Oven

Yield: 12 eggs or 6 portions (2 eggs per portion)

Prep Time: 5 minutes

Cook Time: 20 minutes

Why use the oven to hard-boil eggs? First, it leaves the stovetop free for the preparation of other foods, and second, there is minimal cleanup. Hard-boiled eggs make the perfect protein-packed snack. They're also a great addition to wraps, sandwiches, and salads (see the Tomato, Egg, and Lentil Bowls on page 84).

12 large eggs

4 to 5 cups (950 to 1,180 ml) cold water

8 or 9 ice cubes

1. Preheat the oven to 350°F (180°C). Place 1 egg in each cup of a 12-cup muffin tin or two 6-cup muffin tins.

2. Place the muffin tin(s) on the middle rack of the oven and bake for 20 minutes.

3. Remove from the oven and let the eggs sit while you fill a large bowl with the cold water and ice.

4. Plunge the baked eggs into the ice water, adding more water if the eggs are not completely covered. Let the eggs sit in the ice water for about 10 minutes.

5. Place 2 eggs each, peeled or unpeeled, into 6 containers. Store in the refrigerator for up to 1 week.

PRO PREP TIPS

* Slight brown spots may appear on the shells while cooking, but this will not affect the insides of the eggs.

* Oven temperatures can vary; therefore, the eggs may need to cook 5 more minutes. Test 1 egg at 20 minutes and gauge your cooking time from there. Once you know the exact timing based on your oven temperature, you will always have perfectly cooked eggs.

Cheesy Egg Bites

My clients love this meal-prep idea for their entire family because the ingredients can be changed based on the taste preferences in their homes. Here are some of the combos I like to use: mushroom, spinach, and goat cheese; roasted red peppers and feta cheese; and pizza flavored (pepperoni, tomato, and mozzarella with basil and oregano seasonings).

Yield: 12 egg cups or 4 portions (3 cups per portion)

Prep Time: 10 minutes

Cook Time: 20 minutes

Nonstick cooking spray (olive, coconut, or avocado oil)

10 large eggs

¼ cup (60 ml) milk (dairy, soy, or nut)

Onion powder, to taste

Italian seasoning, to taste

Himalayan pink salt, to taste

Freshly ground black pepper, to taste

3 medium bell peppers (any color), diced

1 cup (75 g) finely chopped broccoli florets

¼ cup (30 g) shredded cheddar cheese

1. Preheat the oven to 375°F (190°C). Grease a 12-cup muffin tin or two 6-cup muffin tins with the cooking spray. Set aside.

2. In a large bowl, whisk together the eggs, milk, onion powder, Italian seasoning, salt, and black pepper.

3. Equally divide the bell peppers, broccoli, and cheese among the muffin cups.

4. Pour the egg mixture over the top of the vegetables, filling each cup three-quarters full.

5. Bake for 20 to 25 minutes, until the egg cups set and a toothpick inserted into the center of a cup comes out clean. Remove from the oven and let cool slightly before taking the cups out of the tins.

6. Place 3 egg cups each into 4 containers. Store in the refrigerator for up to 5 days or in the freezer for up to 3 months. To reheat, warm the egg cups in the oven at 325°F (170°C) for 6 to 7 minutes until heated through. If using the microwave, prick 1 or 2 egg cups with a fork, cover, and heat for 30 to 40 seconds.

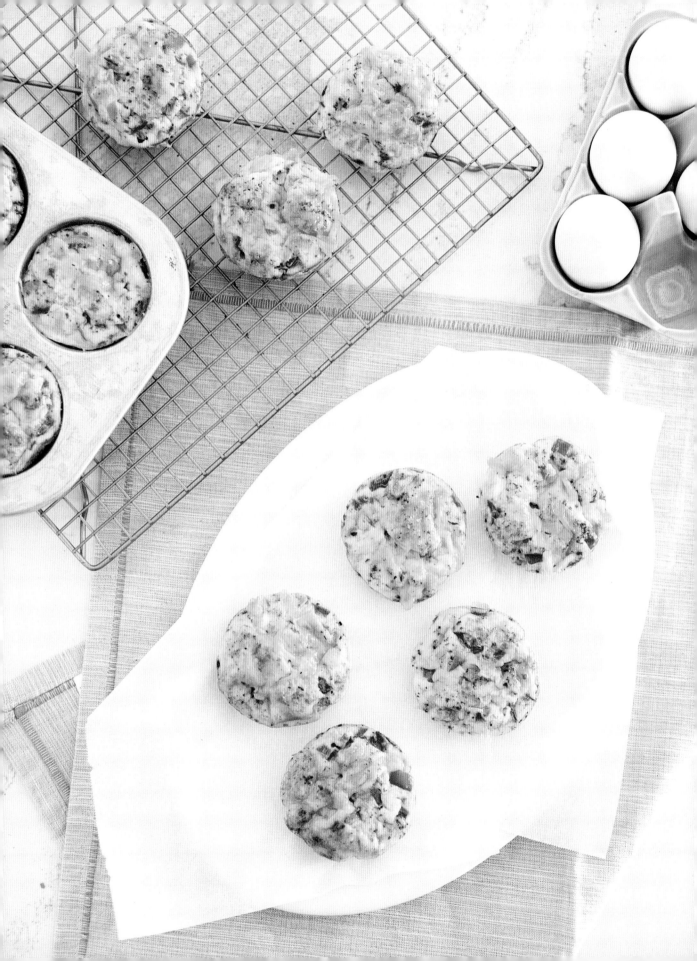

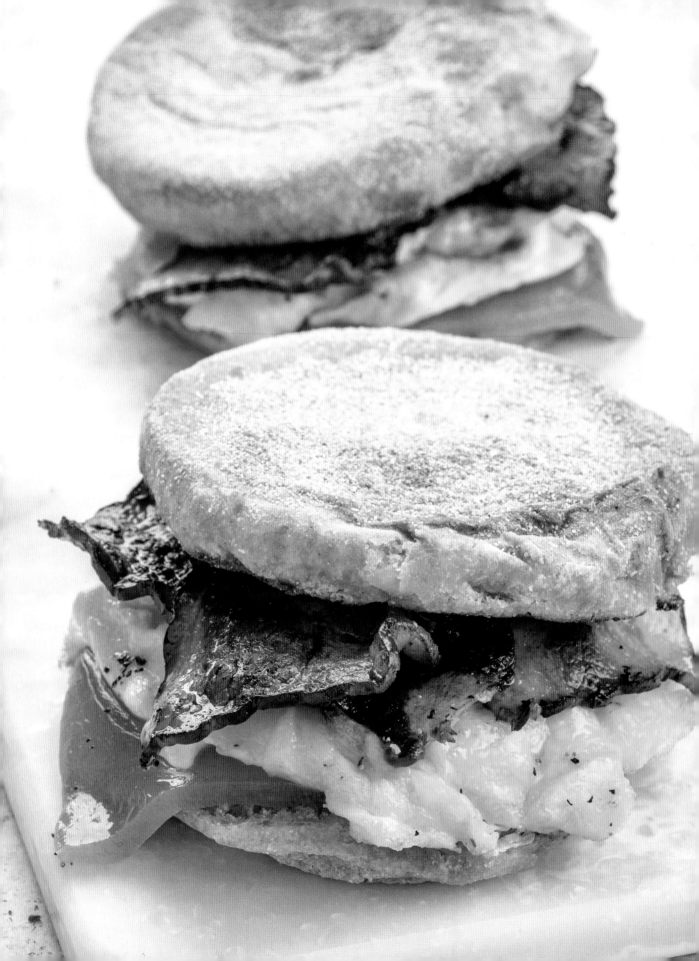

Egg and Cheese English Muffin Sandwiches

Skip the fast food line and make this breakfast classic at home. You can reheat these egg sandwiches quickly and easily in the microwave—perfect for those busy mornings!

Yield: 6 portions
Prep Time: 10 minutes
Cook Time: 15 minutes

Nonstick cooking spray (olive, coconut, or avocado oil)

6 large eggs

1 tablespoon (15 ml) dried oregano

Sea salt or Himalayan pink salt, to taste

Freshly ground black pepper, to taste

6 slices turkey bacon (optional)

6 whole wheat English muffins, sliced in half

6 slices Monterey Jack or cheddar cheese

1. Preheat the oven to 350°F (180°C). Grease a jumbo muffin tin or 6 ramekins with the cooking spray.

2. Crack 1 egg into each muffin cup or ramekin and beat slightly with a fork, avoiding contact with the muffin tin or ramekin. Season the eggs with the oregano, salt, and black pepper.

3. Bake the eggs for 12 to 15 minutes, or until fully set. Remove from the oven and let the eggs cool, 5 to 6 minutes. Run a knife around the edges of the muffin cups or ramekins to remove the eggs.

4. While the eggs are baking, cook the turkey bacon (if using) per the package directions.

5. To assemble the sandwiches, layer one-half of each English muffin with 1 cooked egg, 1 slice of cheese, and 1 slice of turkey bacon (if using). Top with the other half of the English muffin.

6. Individually wrap the sandwiches in aluminum foil and store in the refrigerator for up to 4 days, or wrap in plastic wrap or freezer bags and place in the freezer for up to 3 months. To reheat, remove the foil or plastic wrap and place in the microwave until warmed, 1 to 2 minutes. If frozen, microwave the sandwich on the defrost setting for 2½ to 3 minutes.

Overnight Oats

Overnight oats aren't actually a "new" thing. They are more of a rediscovery of a recipe called bircher muesli that was developed in the early 1900s, and it was love at first taste for me. Oats are loaded with goodness, including vitamins, minerals, and fiber. Any variety of oats will work with this recipe (quick oats, rolled oats, and steel-cut oats). You may have to experiment a little (as Goldilocks did) before you find your perfect texture; the less liquid, the thicker your overnight oats will be. Once you've mastered that, all you need to do is have fun creating your own combinations of add-ins.

Yield: 4 or 5 portions

Prep Time: 10 minutes (plus overnight refrigeration)

1 part base: rolled oats

1 part cold liquid: water, dairy milk (any variety), cashew milk, coconut milk, almond milk, or soy milk

Suggested toppings: raspberries, chopped apple, kiwi, grapes, pear, plum, peaches, figs, melon, banana

Add-ins: chia seeds, hemp hearts (shelled), raisins, chopped nuts, coconut, sunflower seeds, granola, Greek yogurt, vanilla or almond extract, protein powder, cinnamon, nutmeg, pumpkin spice

1. Prep 4 or 5 half-pint (8 ounces, or 227 g) Mason jars at a time. Add the oats to the jars, then pour in an equal amount of cold liquid and stir well. (If using chia seeds, add them in this step.)

2. Refrigerate overnight. Add additional liquid in the morning (if desired). Top with your choice of fruit and add-ins before eating. If you are taking the jar to go, toss the add-ins on top and then mix before eating.

3. Store in the refrigerator for up to 5 days.

PRO PREP TIP

Chia seeds will soak up some of the liquid when added to the oats. Make sure to have some additional cold liquid on hand when you are ready to enjoy the oats and add enough for your desired consistency.

Chia Seed Pudding

This easy, healthy, and delicious pudding is great on its own or with toppings. And you can enjoy it as a breakfast at home or take it to go for a satisfying snack. Here are some of my favorite topping combos: sliced banana and coconut flakes; sliced peaches and shaved ginger; blueberries and sliced strawberries; halved seedless green grapes and ground flaxseed; and peanut butter and dark chocolate chips.

Yield: 4 portions

Prep Time: 10 minutes
(plus 2 hours refrigeration)

1 cup (240 ml) light (reduced fat) coconut milk (from a can)

3 cups (700 ml) milk (dairy or unsweetened nut milk)

10 to 12 tablespoons (60 to 72 g) chia seeds

2 teaspoons (10 ml) pure vanilla extract

4 teaspoons (20 ml) pure maple syrup, or to taste

½ teaspoon ground cinnamon

1. Place all the ingredients into a large bowl (preferably one with a pouring spout) or large glass measuring cup and whisk together.

2. Equally pour the mixture into 4 half-pint (8 ounces, or 227 g) Mason jars and secure the lids.

3. Refrigerate for at least 2 hours to thicken, stirring occasionally. You want the mixture to have a pudding consistency. If the pudding still seems thin at the 2-hour mark, add more chia seeds, 1 tablespoon (6 g) at a time. Stir and let sit in the refrigerator for 20 minutes after each addition.

4. Store in the refrigerator for up to 4 days. When ready to enjoy, add any toppings to the pudding.

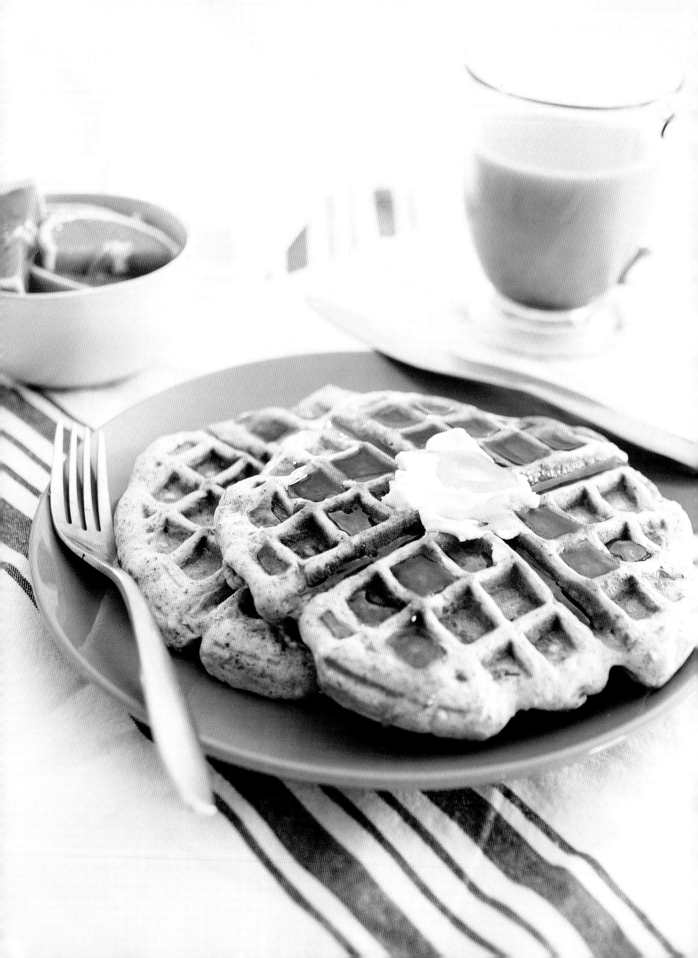

Apple Cinnamon Waffles

Yield: 4 to 6 portions
(1 waffle per portion)

Prep Time: 20 minutes

Cook Time: Varies depending
on waffle iron

I'm pretty new to the waffle game, but once I realized they would work for meal prep, I was hooked. There are so many ways to make waffles your own, from the filling to the toppings—there is no need to stick to butter and syrup when you can keep it healthy with berries or seeds. Boost the protein with Greek yogurt or nut butter.

2 cups (240 g) flour (gluten-free or whole wheat)

2 tablespoons (30 ml) flaxseed meal

1 tablespoon (15 ml) baking powder

1 teaspoon ground cinnamon

¼ teaspoon Himalayan pink salt

1½ cups (350 ml) almond milk, plus more if needed

2 large eggs

¾ cup (180 g) unsweetened applesauce

1 teaspoon pure vanilla extract

1 tablespoon (15 ml) pure maple syrup

1 apple of choice, diced (optional)

¾ cup (90 g) chopped pecans (optional)

PRO PREP TIP

To freeze these waffles, let them cool completely on the cooling rack. Place a square of parchment or wax paper in between each waffle and wrap a stack of waffles in plastic wrap or put into a resealable freezer bag. Store in the freezer for up to 3 months.

1. Since waffle irons can vary, follow the instructions included with your iron for preheating, prepping the iron (cooking spray or oil may be suggested), and cooking.

2. In a large bowl, combine the flour, flaxseed meal, baking powder, cinnamon, and pink salt.

3. In a medium bowl, whisk together the 1½ cups (350 ml) almond milk, eggs, applesauce, vanilla, and maple syrup.

4. Add the wet ingredients to the dry ingredients, along with the diced apple (if using) and pecan pieces (if using), and mix together. If the batter is too dry, add more almond milk, 1 tablespoon (15 ml) at a time, and mix.

5. Use a ¾ cup (180 ml) measuring cup to scoop and pour the batter onto the center of the waffle iron. When the waffle is done, slip a rubber spatula underneath the waffle to lift it off the iron. Let cool on a cooling rack. Repeat this step with the remaining batter.

6. Once cool, place each waffle into a container. Store in the refrigerator for up to 5 days. To reheat, warm in the microwave, toaster, or toaster oven.

Berry Vanilla High-Protein Pancakes

Yield: About 9 pancakes or 3 portions (3 pancakes per portion)

Prep Time: 15 minutes

Cook Time: 20 minutes

You don't have to save these pancakes for breakfast; they can act as a filling, healthy midmorning or afternoon snack too! I've been known to eat these pancakes cold, but you can also reheat them.

2 cups (160 g) rolled oats

1¼ cups (295 ml) unsweetened almond milk, plus more if needed

2 scoops vanilla whey protein powder

½ cup (60 g) coconut flour

½ cup (120 g) unsweetened applesauce

1 teaspoon pure vanilla extract

Coconut oil, for cooking

1 cup (75 g) frozen or fresh mixed berries (e.g., raspberries, blueberries, blackberries), for topping

¾ cup (64 g) unsweetened desiccated coconut, for topping (optional)

1. Place the oats, almond milk, protein powder, coconut flour, applesauce, and vanilla (in the order they are listed) into a blender. Blend on low to medium until well combined. If the batter is too thick—doesn't pour easily off a spoon—add more almond milk, 1 tablespoon (15 ml) at a time, and blend until the desired consistency is reached.

2. Heat a large nonstick skillet over medium-high heat. Add enough coconut oil to coat the pan when melted. You may need to cook in batches, so if the pan becomes dry at some point, add a little bit more coconut oil. Slowly pour the batter from the blender onto the skillet, forming circles about the size of the palm of a hand. When the edges of the pancakes start to look dry and bubbles begin to form, 2 to 3 minutes, flip and cook for 1 to 2 more minutes on the other side. Remove from the heat.

3. Place 3 pancakes each into 3 containers, storing the toppings in separate containers. Store in the refrigerator for up to 4 days. To reheat, warm the pancakes in the microwave, toaster, or toaster oven. Top with the berries, warmed for 30 seconds in the microwave if frozen, and coconut (if using).

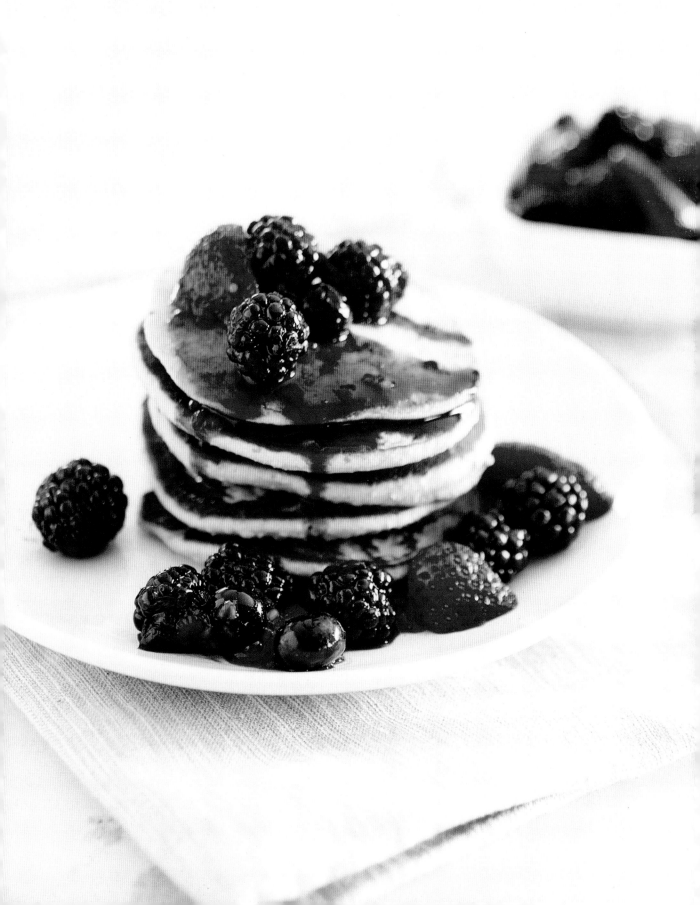

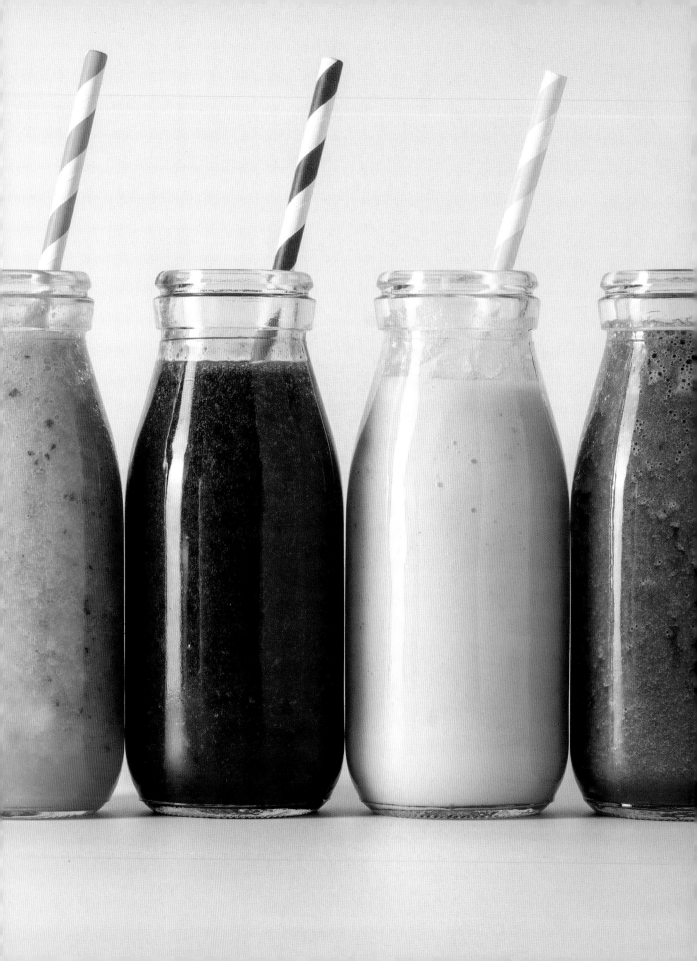

Smoothies

To prep any of these smoothies ahead of time, place all the ingredients (except the protein powder and liquid) into a resealable plastic freezer bag and place in the freezer. Arrange 1 bag for each day of the week. When you are ready to make your smoothie, simply dump the contents of the bag into the blender, add your protein powder and liquid, and blend. Frozen smoothie bags are best used within 6 weeks of preparation.

Yield: 1 portion

Prep Time: 5 minutes

MOCHA MONKEY SMOOTHIE

½ teaspoon instant coffee

½ frozen banana

1 scoop chocolate whey protein powder

1 tablespoon (15 ml) chia seeds

1 tablespoon (14 g) raw almond butter

2 ice cubes

1 cup (240 ml) almond milk (unsweetened vanilla or plain)

HEALTHY BOOSTER SMOOTHIE

1 cup (70 g) baby spinach

½ cup (83 g) chopped pineapple or 1 pineapple spear (fresh or frozen)

Flesh of ⅓ avocado

Juice of ¼ lemon

3 ice cubes

½ teaspoon raw honey

1 tablespoon (15 ml) ground flaxseed

Pinch sea salt

½ cup (120 ml) coconut water

TO MAKE MOCHA MONKEY SMOOTHIE

1. Place all the ingredients (in the order they are listed) into a high-speed blender and blend until smooth, 30 to 60 seconds (depending on your blender).

2. Serve immediately.

TO MAKE HEALTHY BOOSTER SMOOTHIE

1. Place all the ingredients (in the order they are listed) into a high-speed blender and blend until smooth, 30 to 60 seconds (depending on your blender).

2. Serve immediately.

continued

PINEAPPLE-GINGER GREEN SMOOTHIE

1 cup (67 g) kale

½ cup (83 g) chopped pineapple or 1 pineapple spear (fresh or frozen)

¼ green apple

Juice of ½ lemon

1 small slice ginger (approximately ½ teaspoon minced), peeled

½ cup (52 g) chopped cucumber or 1 large cucumber spear

1 scoop hemp protein powder

1 cup (240 ml) coconut milk (unsweetened from a carton)

VERY BERRY SMOOTHIE

½ cup (75 g) frozen mixed berries

¾ cup (50 g) baby spinach

½ cup (120 g) nonfat plain Greek-style yogurt

1 scoop vanilla whey protein powder

1 cup (240 ml) almond milk (unsweetened vanilla or plain)

TO MAKE PINEAPPLE-GINGER GREEN SMOOTHIE

1. Place all the ingredients (in the order they are listed) into a high-speed blender and blend until smooth, 30 to 60 seconds (depending on your blender).

2. Serve immediately.

TO MAKE VERY BERRY SMOOTHIE

1. Place all the ingredients (in the order they are listed) into a high-speed blender and blend until smooth, 30 to 60 seconds (depending on your blender).

2. Serve immediately.

PRO PREP TIP

If you don't have a high-speed blender and are finding it difficult to get rid of leafy chunks when blending, blend the greens with some of the liquid for 30 to 45 seconds before adding the rest of the ingredients. If your ingredients still aren't blending, you may need to remove the blender from the base, give it a shake, and try again. If you are using a high-speed blender, start blending on low speed and slowly increase to the maximum speed.

Chocolate Raspberry Breakfast Quinoa

Yield: 3 or 4 portions

Prep Time: 10 minutes

Cook Time: 25 minutes

Quinoa is a staple food for meal prep—it is easy to cook and keeps well through the week. If this breakfast bowl doesn't get you up in the morning, then I don't know what will!

1 cup (173 g) quinoa, rinsed

2 cups (475 ml) coconut milk (from a carton), plus more for serving

1 teaspoon raw honey

2 tablespoons (30 ml) raw cacao powder or unsweetened cocoa powder

½ teaspoon pure vanilla extract

½ teaspoon ground cinnamon

Pinch Himalayan pink salt

¼ cup (23 g) sliced almonds, for topping (optional)

1 cup (120 g) raspberries, for topping (optional)

1. In a medium pot with a lid, combine the quinoa, coconut milk, and honey. Bring to a boil, reduce the heat, cover, and cook at a slow simmer for about 15 minutes, stirring frequently, until the quinoa is cooked through.

2. Stir in the cocoa, vanilla, cinnamon, and pink salt until well combined. Remove from the heat.

3. Equally divide the quinoa into 3 or 4 containers or Mason jars, storing the toppings (if using) in separate containers. Store in the refrigerator for up to 4 days. To reheat, add a splash of coconut milk, stir, and heat in the microwave for 30 to 40 seconds. Top with the almonds (if using) and raspberries (if using).

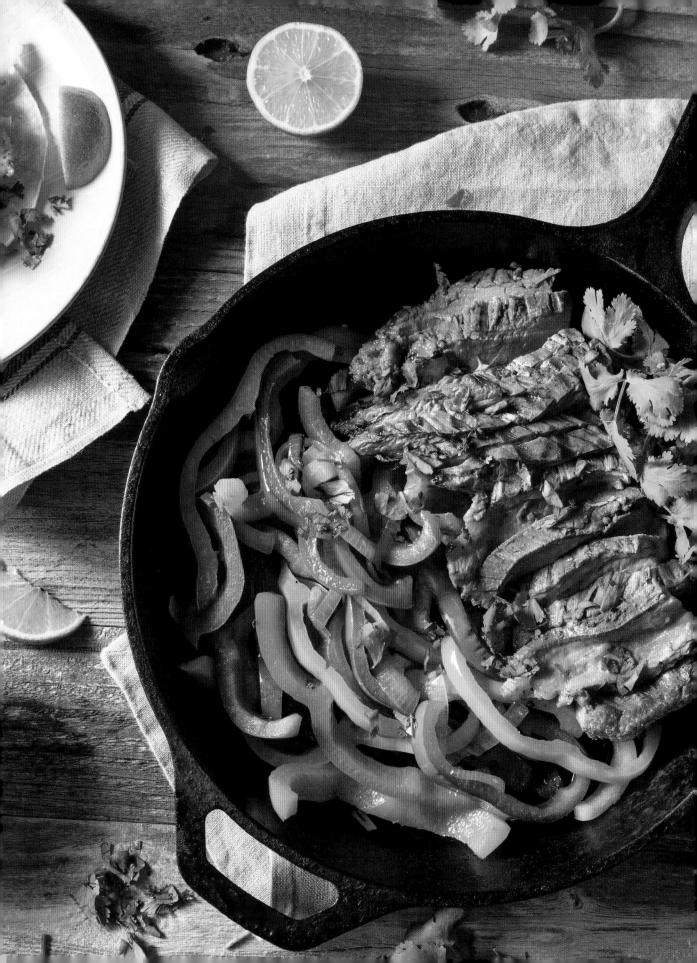

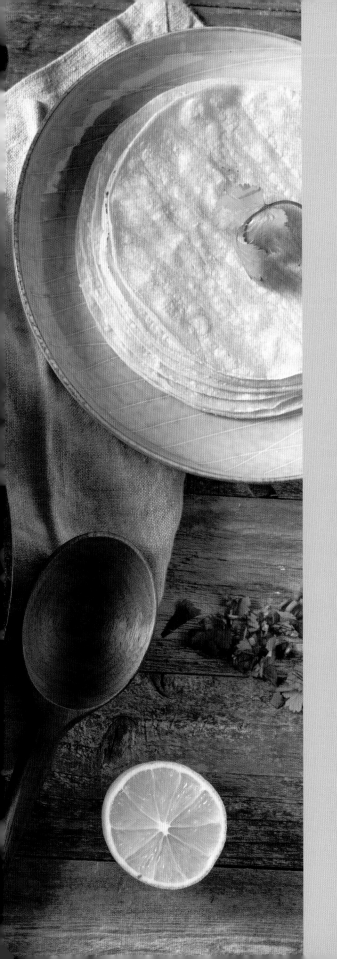

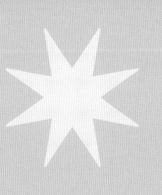

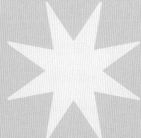

MAINS

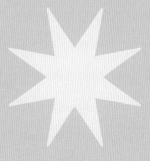

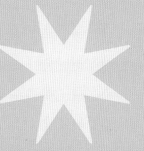

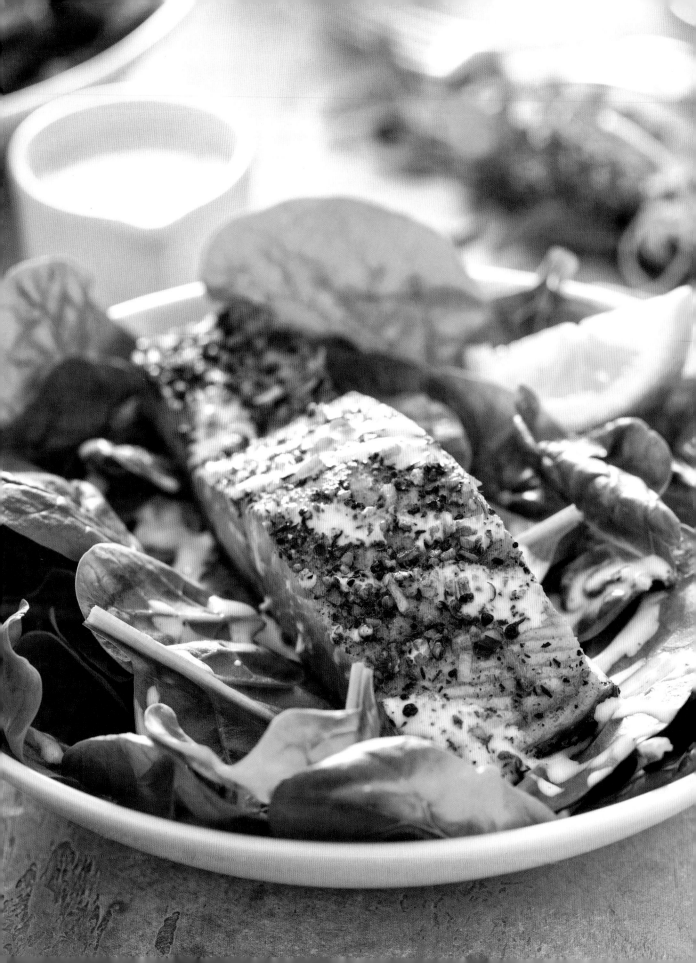

Baked Salmon with Paprika and Lemon

Yield: 4 portions

Prep Time: 10 minutes

Cook Time: 15 minutes

This salmon is delicious when sliced and served cold on top of the Superfood Green Salad (page 63).

1 tablespoon (15 ml) extra-virgin olive oil, plus more for drizzling

1 teaspoon smoked paprika

1 teaspoon garlic powder

1 teaspoon Himalayan pink salt

½ teaspoon freshly ground black pepper

1 lemon, zested and juiced

4 wild salmon fillets, with skin (each 6 ounces, or 170 g, and 1 inch, or 2.5 cm, thick)

1. Preheat the oven to 400°F (200°C). Line a large, rimmed baking sheet with aluminum foil, then drizzle a little olive oil to coat the foil.

2. In a small bowl, whisk together the 1 tablespoon (15 ml) olive oil, paprika, garlic powder, pink salt, black pepper, and lemon zest.

3. Place the salmon fillets, skin sides down, on the prepared baking sheet. Spoon out the lemon-spice mixture and spread onto the fillets.

4. Bake for 15 to 20 minutes, or until the salmon is fully cooked and easily flakes with a fork. Remove from the oven and drizzle the salmon with the lemon juice. Let the salmon rest and cool on the baking sheet.

5. Place each fillet into a container and store in the refrigerator for up to 4 days. Eat cold or reheat in the microwave for 30 seconds per fillet or warm in the oven at 350°F (180°C) for 5 minutes.

Ultimate Black Bean Burgers

You'll never want to eat a frozen veggie burger again after tasting this burger made with clean ingredients.

Yield: 4 or 5 portions (1 burger per portion)

Prep Time: 15 minutes

Cook Time: 10 minutes

2 cups (500 g) canned black beans, rinsed, drained, and patted dry with a paper towel

1 cup (80 g) rolled oats

1 cup (110 g) shredded carrot

½ cup (80 g) chopped yellow or white onion

2 garlic cloves, minced

¼ cup (22 g) chopped cabbage

1 medium tomato, chopped

2 large eggs

2 to 3 tablespoons (30 to 45 ml) extra-virgin olive oil, divided

½ teaspoon sea salt

½ teaspoon freshly ground black pepper

½ teaspoon smoked paprika

½ teaspoon onion powder

Suggested toppings: lettuce, sliced onion, sliced tomato, avocado, roasted red peppers, mustard, hummus

4 or 5 thin whole-grain buns (optional)

1. Place the beans, oats, carrot, onion, garlic, cabbage, tomato, eggs, 1 tablespoon (15 ml) of the olive oil, sea salt, black pepper, paprika, and onion powder into a food processor and pulse until a mixture resembling the consistency of crumbled meat is reached. Do not overmix.

2. Mold the mixture into 4 or 5 equal-size patties, about the size of a palm of a hand, and place on parchment paper. (Note: If the mixture is slightly sticky, wet your hands with cold water and continue.)

3. Heat the remaining 1 to 2 tablespoons (15 to 30 ml) olive oil in a large skillet over medium heat. Cook the patties for 5 minutes on each side, or until golden brown.

4. Place each burger into a container and store in the refrigerator for up to 4 days, storing any toppings and the buns (if using) in separate containers. To reheat, microwave for 30 seconds or warm in a skillet with a drizzle of olive oil. Assemble with the toppings.

PRO PREP TIP

To freeze, place the cooked burgers on a parchment-lined baking sheet and freeze for a couple hours. Once frozen, transfer them to a freezer bag. Reheat after thawing.

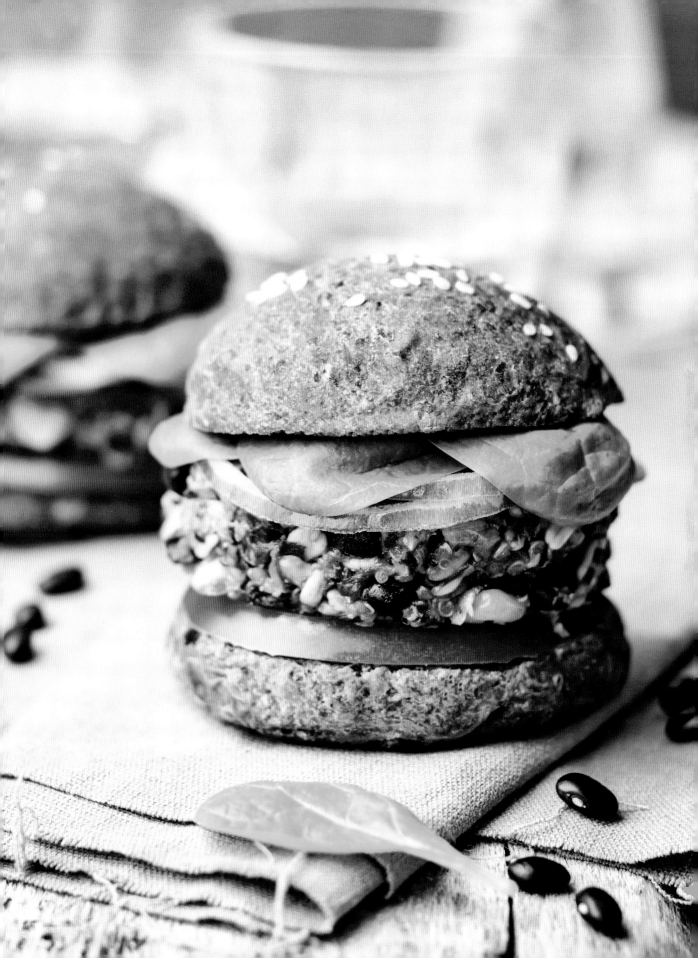

Chicken and Bacon Club Wraps

Wraps are the perfect bring-to-work meal; this no-fuss, no-muss meal is easy to pack (no utensils needed).

Yield: 4 portions

Prep Time: 15 minutes

Cook Time: 15 minutes

CHICKEN

3 boneless and skinless chicken breasts (6 ounces, or 170 g, each), sliced in half lengthwise

Himalayan pink salt, to taste

Freshly ground black pepper, to taste

1 tablespoon (15 ml) extra-virgin olive oil

WRAPS

4 large (10 inches, or 25 cm, each) whole wheat tortillas

2 teaspoons yellow mustard, divided

4 slices turkey bacon, cooked according to package instructions

8 leaves romaine lettuce

2 beefsteak tomatoes, sliced

1. **To make the chicken:** Season the chicken breasts with the pink salt and black pepper. Heat the olive oil in a large skillet over medium-high heat for 30 seconds. Add the chicken to the skillet without overlapping the pieces. Flip each chicken breast over once the underside is golden brown, about 6 minutes per side. To check for doneness, slice through one of the chicken breasts to see that the meat is white and the juices run clear. Remove the chicken from the pan and let cool on a clean cutting board, 6 to 7 minutes.

2. When the chicken has cooled, diagonally slice it into strips. You can begin to assemble the wraps or store the chicken strips in an airtight container in the refrigerator for up to 4 days.

3. **To assemble the wraps:** Lay out the tortillas on a clean surface. Spread about ½ teaspoon of mustard on each tortilla, leaving a ½-inch (13 mm) border around the edges. Top each tortilla with one-quarter of the sliced chicken, 1 strip of the turkey bacon, 2 leaves of the lettuce, and the tomato slices.

4. To roll the wrap, start at the edge closest to you, fold the tortilla up slightly with your thumbs, fold the sides in with your fingers, and continue to tuck and roll to create a burrito-like wrap. Repeat with the remaining tortillas.

5. Wrap each wrap in aluminum foil and store in the refrigerator for up to 2 days. If you are making more than 2 days' worth of wraps, store the toppings separately for up to 5 days and assemble the wraps the day of eating.

Spinach Fettuccine with Turkey Bolognese

Yield: 6 to 8 portions

Prep Time: 10 minutes

Cook Time: 25 minutes

I was excited to add turkey Bolognese as a "foodprepable" recipe. My Instagram community voted this recipe in, so I guess you could say it's a fan favorite. No need to simmer this sauce for hours to get the rich and delicious taste that Bolognese is known for—you'll be twirling your pasta around your fork in less than 40 minutes.

1 tablespoon (15 ml) extra-virgin olive oil

1 small red onion, finely chopped

2 garlic cloves, minced

1 large carrot, peeled and finely chopped

1 celery rib, finely chopped

3 tablespoons (45 g) tomato paste

½ teaspoon Himalayan pink salt

½ teaspoon freshly ground black pepper

1 teaspoon Italian seasoning

1 pound (454 g) lean ground turkey

1 can (28 ounces, or 794 g) whole peeled tomatoes (with juices)

10 ounces (280 g) fresh spinach fettuccine

1. Heat the olive oil in a large skillet with a lid over medium heat for 30 seconds.

2. Add the onion and garlic, and cook and stir until the onion is translucent, about 5 minutes. Add the carrot and celery, and cook and stir until the vegetables are tender, about 5 minutes.

3. Add the tomato paste, pink salt, black pepper, and Italian seasoning, and stir to combine the ingredients. Add the ground turkey and tomatoes. Reduce the heat to medium-low, cover, and gently simmer for 15 minutes, stirring often. When the turkey is fully cooked (no longer pink inside or a meat thermometer reaches 165°F, or 75°C), turn the heat off but leave the sauce in the skillet.

4. While the sauce is simmering, cook the fettuccine in a large pot of boiling salted water for 2 to 3 minutes, until al dente. Reserve ½ cup (120 ml) of the cooking liquid, then drain the pasta.

5. Add the pasta to the sauce and toss to coat, adding enough of the reserved cooking liquid to moisten if needed.

6. Equally divide the pasta into 6 to 8 containers. Store in the refrigerator for up to 4 or 5 days. To reheat, warm in a skillet over medium-high heat for 5 to 6 minutes, stirring frequently. If using the microwave, warm for 2 minutes, stirring halfway through the cooking time.

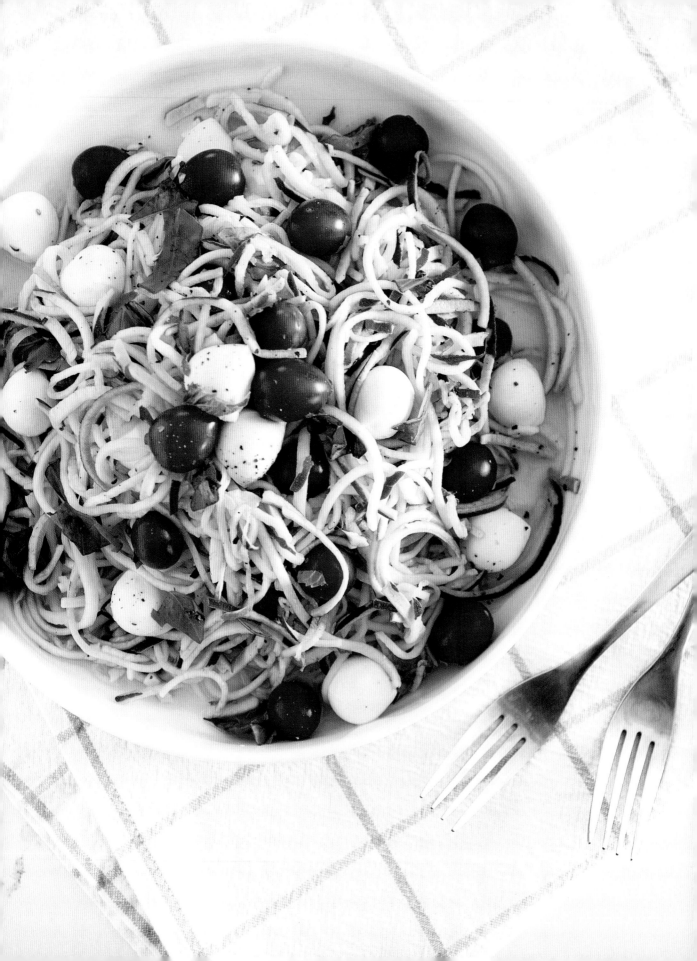

Zucchini Noodles Caprese-Style

Yield: 4 portions

Prep Time: 20 minutes

You can create zucchini noodles with a countertop spiralizer, a handheld spiralizer, or a *Y* vegetable peeler. If using a countertop spiralizer, cut off both ends of the zucchini, position it in the spiralizer, and turn the handle to make a beautiful pile of curly "noodles." With a handheld spiralizer, use it like a large pencil sharpener. Run a *Y* or julienne vegetable peeler down the entire length of the zucchini to create ribbon-like strands.

3 medium zucchini, unpeeled and spiralized

2 pints (550 g) cherry tomatoes

16 mini bocconcini (mozzarella cheese balls; if you can't find bocconcini, a ball of fresh mozzarella cheese cut into cubes will work)

½ cup (20 g) roughly chopped fresh basil leaves

¼ cup (60 ml) balsamic vinegar

2 tablespoons (30 ml) extra-virgin olive oil

Dried oregano, to taste

Himalayan pink salt, to taste

Freshly ground black pepper, to taste

2 cooked boneless and skinless chicken breasts (6 to 8 ounces, or 170 to 227 g, each), sliced in half lengthwise (optional)

1. To a large bowl, add the spiralized zucchini, tomatoes, cheese, and basil.

2. Drizzle the vinegar and olive oil on top, and season with the oregano, salt, and black pepper. Toss to combine.

3. Equally divide the salad into 4 containers and top with the chicken (if using). Store in the refrigerator for up to 4 days.

PRO PREP TIP

If you'd like to keep the salad and dressing separate, equally divide the spiralized zucchini, tomatoes, cheese, basil, and sliced chicken (if using) into the 4 containers and store the olive oil, vinegar, and spices together in small containers. Dress the salad when you are ready to enjoy it.

Stuffed Sweet Potatoes

This irresistible combo is a favorite with my family and my clients! You will have leftover "stuffing," so enjoy it on its own or add it to another tasty meal. I love to mix it with eggs for a super-satisfying breakfast; simply add it to the pan when cooking your eggs.

Yield: 4 portions
Prep Time: 15 minutes
Cook Time: 1 hour

4 medium sweet potatoes, unpeeled

1 teaspoon olive oil

2 boneless and skinless chicken breasts (6 ounces, or 170 g, each)

3 cups (210 g) finely chopped broccoli florets

¼ cup (40 g) diced white onion

½ teaspoon sea salt

½ teaspoon garlic powder

½ teaspoon chili powder

Dash cayenne pepper (optional)

¼ cup (30 g) grated low-fat cheddar cheese

1. Preheat the oven to 400°F (200°C).

2. Poke the sweet potatoes with a fork a few times and place them in a baking dish or on a large baking sheet. Drizzle the olive oil into the bottom of another baking dish with a lid and place the chicken breasts into the dish.

3. Bake the sweet potatoes for 50 to 60 minutes, and bake the chicken, covered, for 25 to 30 minutes (if you don't have a lid, cover securely with aluminum foil).

4. Meanwhile, place the broccoli into a large microwave-safe bowl. Add 2 tablespoons (30 ml) of water, cover with a plate, and steam in the microwave for 3 minutes.

5. When the chicken is cooked, check it for doneness; slice through one of the chicken breasts to see that the meat is white and the juices run clear. With 2 forks, shred all the chicken. Add the shredded chicken to the bowl with the steamed broccoli.

6. When the sweet potatoes are done, cut a slit in the top of each potato. Scoop out most of the flesh, leaving the skins intact. Add the flesh to the bowl with the broccoli and chicken. Add the onion, sea salt, garlic powder, chili powder, and cayenne (if using) to the bowl. Mix the ingredients until well combined.

7. Scoop this mixture into the potato skins. Sprinkle the cheese on top of each potato. Place each potato into a container and store in the refrigerator for up to 5 days. To reheat, microwave for 1½ to 2½ minutes or warm in the oven at 350°F (180°C) for about 20 minutes.

Superfood Green Salad

Yield: 4 portions

Prep Time: 10 minutes

The Basic Salad Dressing (page 139) is the perfect way to amplify all the goodness in this healthy dish.

3 cups (555 g) cooked quinoa (red or white)

6 cups (180 g) baby spinach

2 cups (60 g) sprouts (broccoli, pea, sunflower, or alfalfa)

2 medium English cucumbers, chopped

4 teaspoons (24 g) chia seeds

4 teaspoons (12 g) sunflower seeds

4 teaspoons (12 g) pumpkin seeds

Chopped fresh parsley, for topping

1 recipe Basic Salad Dressing (page 139), equally divided into 4 small containers

1. Place the quinoa, spinach, sprouts, cucumbers, and chia, sunflower, and pumpkin seeds in a large bowl, and toss until combined.

2. Equally divide the salad into 4 containers and top with the parsley. Store in the refrigerator for up to 4 days. When ready to enjoy, pour the salad dressing over the salad and toss thoroughly to combine.

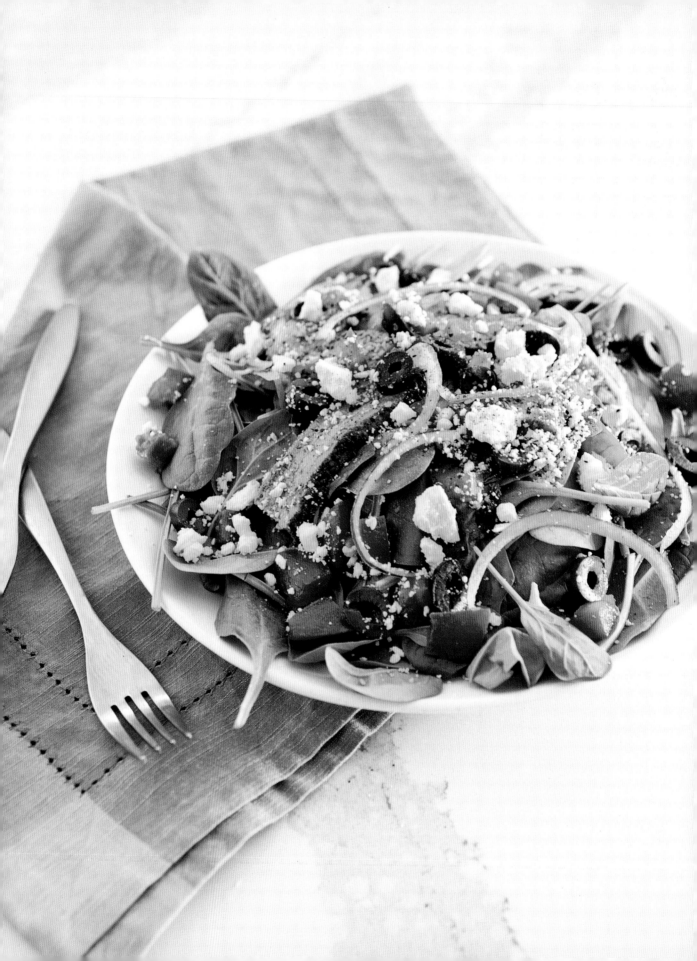

Mediterranean Steak Salad

Yield: 4 portions

Prep Time: 30 minutes

Cook Time: 10 minutes

The healthy fats, protein, and vegetables make this salad a perfect lunch or dinner that is satisfying and delicious. You can eat the steak cold or warm, which makes it great for prep!

DRESSING

¼ cup (60 ml) extra-virgin olive oil

2 tablespoons (30 ml) red wine vinegar

Fresh oregano, to taste

Himalayan pink salt, to taste

Freshly ground black pepper, to taste

SALAD

2 boneless New York strip steaks (10 ounces, or 283 g, each)

Himalayan pink salt, to taste

Freshly ground black pepper, to taste

4 cups (120 g) leafy greens (such as spinach, spring mix, or endive)

4 Roma tomatoes, chopped

8 kalamata olives, drained, pitted, and chopped

½ red onion, separated into rings

1 cup (150 g) crumbled feta cheese

1. **To make the dressing:** Place all the dressing ingredients into a Mason jar or sealable container and secure with the lid. Shake to combine. Equally divide the dressing into 4 small containers.

2. **To make the salad:** Sprinkle both sides of the steaks with the pink salt and black pepper, and let come to room temperature before cooking.

3. Preheat a grill or large nonstick skillet over medium heat. Place the steaks on the grill/in the pan and cook for 4 to 5 minutes per side, or until desired doneness. Remove the steaks from the grill/pan and let rest on a cutting board for 5 minutes. Thinly slice.

4. Equally divide the greens, tomatoes, olives, onion, and cheese into 4 containers and top the salad with the steak slices. Store in the refrigerator for up to 2 days. If you prefer the steak warmed, heat only the steak in the microwave for 45 seconds. When ready to enjoy, shake the dressing, pour onto the salad, and combine. If you are making more than 2 days' worth of salad and steak, store the steak in separate containers from the salad for up to 4 days.

Thai Bowls with Peanut Sauce

If you ask me, the peanut sauce is what makes this dish so good!

Yield: 4 portions

Prep Time: 15 minutes

PEANUT SAUCE

¼ cup (60 g) natural creamy peanut butter

2 tablespoons (30 ml) soy sauce

1 tablespoon (15 ml) rice wine vinegar

1 teaspoon freshly grated ginger

1 teaspoon raw honey (optional)

2 to 3 tablespoons (30 to 45 ml) warm water

BOWLS

2 cups (320 g) cooked brown rice

1 teaspoon sesame oil

1 bag (16 ounces, or 454 g) shelled edamame (thawed if using frozen)

1 large red bell pepper, diced

½ large seedless cucumber, diced

1 medium-to-large carrot, julienned

4 scallions, chopped, plus more for topping

¼ cup (10 g) roughly chopped Thai basil leaves

2 tablespoons (16 g) sesame seeds (white or black), for topping

1. **To make the peanut sauce:** Place all the peanut sauce ingredients into a Mason jar or sealable container and secure with the lid. Shake to combine. Add warm water, 1 tablespoon (15 ml) at a time, to thin the dressing to desired consistency.

2. Equally divide the sauce into 4 small containers. Store in the refrigerator for up to 5 days. The sauce may need to be reheated to make it pourable. Simply pop the jar (without the lid) into the microwave for 20 seconds, stir and pour.

3. **To make the bowls:** Drizzle the cooked rice with the sesame oil and set aside to cool (if the rice isn't already cooled). To a large bowl, add the edamame, bell pepper, cucumber, carrot, scallions, and basil, and toss until well combined.

4. To assemble the bowls, equally divide the rice into 4 containers, followed by the vegetable mixture, storing the toppings in separate containers. Top each portion with a sprinkle of sesame seeds and some chopped scallion. Store in the refrigerator for up to 5 days. When you are ready to enjoy, pour the desired amount of peanut sauce over the vegetables and rice, and combine.

Pesto Tilapia

You can adapt this recipe to suit almost any type of fish. Red snapper and catfish, among other types of fish, have a similar nutrient profile and also a mild taste, which is the perfect pairing with the freshness of the pesto.

Yield: 4 portions

Prep Time: 10 minutes

Cook Time: 10 minutes

2 tablespoons (30 ml) olive oil

4 tilapia fillets (each 6 to 8 ounces, or 170 to 227 g)

1 teaspoon sea salt

1 teaspoon freshly ground black pepper

½ cup (120 g) Pesto (page 137)

½ cup (50 g) freshly grated Parmesan cheese, divided

½ lemon

1. Heat the olive oil in a large skillet over medium heat until sizzling.

2. Place the tilapia in the pan without overlapping the fillets and season each fillet with the sea salt and black pepper.

3. Cook the fillets for 3 to 4 minutes on one side then flip them over. Smear the pesto on the fillets and cook for 3 to 4 more minutes, until the undersides turn a nice golden brown. Sprinkle the Parmesan cheese and squeeze lemon juice onto the cooked fillets.

4. Place each fillet into a container. Store in the refrigerator for up to 4 days. To reheat, microwave for 45 to 60 seconds, warm in a skillet over medium heat for 4 to 5 minutes, or place in the oven at 375°F (190°C) for 4 to 5 minutes.

Vegetable and Tofu Skewers

Yield: 6 to 9 skewers or 2 or 3 portions (3 skewers per portion)

Prep Time: 30 minutes

Cook Time: 20 minutes

You can enjoy this vegetarian delight on its own or pair it with your favorite grain. Cook these skewers on a grill, on a grill pan on the stove, or under an oven broiler. If you are using wood skewers, you must soak them in water for at least 30 minutes before using.

2 packages (14 ounces, or 396 g, each) extra-firm tofu

2 tablespoons (30 ml) tamari

3 tablespoons (45 ml) barbecue sauce

6 to 9 skewers

2 large zucchini, cut into bite-size pieces

1 large red bell pepper, cut into bite-size pieces

1 large yellow bell pepper, cut into bite-size pieces

1 large red onion, cut into bite-size pieces

2 cups (300 g) cherry tomatoes

1. Remove the tofu from its packaging and drain any liquid. Set the blocks of tofu onto folded paper towels (you may want to put a plate underneath the paper towels to catch excess liquid). Set another folded paper towel on top of each block. Put a plate or small cutting board on top of the tofu and press down firmly to remove the liquid.

2. Remove the tofu from the paper towels and place on a cutting board. Cut the tofu into 1-inch (2.5 cm) cubes and place in a large resealable plastic bag. Pour the tamari and barbecue sauce into the resealable bag, securely seal the bag, and shake to coat. Let the tofu marinate in the refrigerator for at least 10 minutes and up to 30 minutes.

3. Thread the marinated tofu, zucchini, bell peppers, onion, and cherry tomatoes, alternating between the tofu cubes and vegetables, onto the skewers.

4. To cook the skewers, choose your preferred method for cooking (see the recipe note above) and cook for 6 to 12 minutes, depending on your oven, stovetop, or grill. Turn often to brown each side before removing from the heat.

5. Wrap each skewer in aluminum foil after cooling and store in the refrigerator for up to 4 days. Alternatively, you can remove the pieces from the skewer and store them in airtight containers for up to 4 days. Reheat the skewers in the oven at 350°F (180°C) for 4 to 5 minutes.

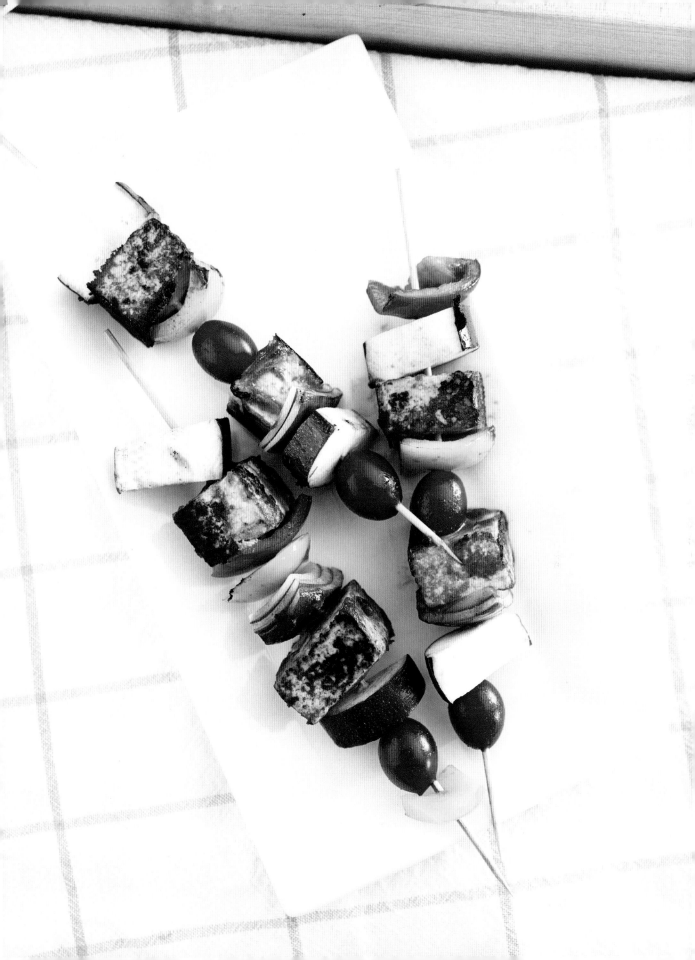

Falafel Bowls

When my craving for warm and savory Middle Eastern food hits, I comply. Instead of deep-frying these gems, I pan-fry them in just a little oil to cut down on the calories but to keep that yummy crunch of the falafel. This bowl is an alternative to the classic pita, but you can use the falafel any way you like.

Yield: 12 to 20 falafel or 4 portion (3 to 5 falafel per portion)

Prep Time: 25 minutes (plus overnight soaking)

Cook Time: 10 minutes

FALAFEL

1½ cups (375 g) dried chickpeas

⅓ cup (20 g) chopped fresh parsley

4 garlic cloves, minced

2 shallots, minced

2 tablespoons (30 g) tahini

½ teaspoon ground cumin

¼ teaspoon Himalayan pink salt

¼ teaspoon freshly ground black pepper

3 to 4 tablespoons (24 to 32 g) whole wheat or chickpea flour

Extra-virgin olive oil, for cooking

BOWLS

1 cup (30 g) baby spinach

¾ cup (110 g) diced bell pepper (any color)

¾ cup (90 g) chopped celery

1 tablespoon (15 ml) extra-virgin olive oil

1 tablespoon (15 ml) red wine vinegar

1. **To make the falafel:** Pour the dried chickpeas into a large bowl and add enough cold water until the chickpeas are just covered. Place a clean dish towel over the top of the bowl and let the chickpeas soak overnight on the counter. (Note: If it's warm in your house, you may opt to soak the chickpeas in the refrigerator.) When you're ready to prepare the falafel, drain any liquid from the chickpeas and pat them dry with a paper towel.

2. Add the soaked chickpeas, parsley, garlic, shallots, tahini, cumin, pink salt, and black pepper to a food processor or blender. Pulse to combine and stop to scrape down the sides when needed. When the mixture forms a crumbly dough, start adding the flour, 1 teaspoon at a time, to absorb any wetness. Don't overmix the dough. Test the dough by forming a small ball in your hands; if the dough sticks together and not to your hands, it is done. Refrigerate the dough for about an hour to help the falafel stay together while cooking.

3. When you're ready to cook the falafel, line a baking sheet with parchment paper and a large plate with paper towels. Set aside.

4. Form the falafel dough into balls the size of golf balls and press them onto the parchment-lined baking sheet to flatten slightly.

5. Heat a large skillet over medium heat and add enough olive oil to generously coat the pan, about 2 tablespoons (30 ml). To test to see if the oil is hot enough, sprinkle a drop of water into the pan. If it sizzles/pops, it is ready.

6. Add the falafel balls to the pan. Do not overcrowd. Cook until the underside is golden brown, 3 to 4 minutes, and then, using silicone-handle tongs, turn them over one by one, cooking them for 3 to 4 more minutes. Remove from the skillet and transfer them to the paper towel–lined plate to absorb any oil.

7. Once cooked, store the falafel in an airtight container in the refrigerator for up to 4 days or freeze them in freezer bags for up to 3 months.

8. **To assemble the bowls:** Equally divide the spinach, bell pepper, and celery into 4 containers, storing 3 to 5 falafel each in 4 separate containers for up to 5 days. You can enjoy the falafel cold or warm; to reheat, microwave for 30 seconds or warm in the oven at 375°F (190°C) for 5 to 6 minutes. When ready to enjoy, drizzle the salad with the olive oil and vinegar, and toss to coat the vegetables. Top with the falafel.

PRO PREP TIPS

* If you are short on time, you can use canned chickpeas. Two cans (15 ounces, or 425 g, each), drained and rinsed, will give you the same quantity of beans needed for the recipe.

* Making falafel from scratch can be tricky. If the balls are not binding together, add flour, 1 tablespoon (8 g) at a time, to your mixture, until you can easily press it into balls or patties. Warming the mixture in the microwave for 20-second increments before rolling into balls can also help bind the mixture.

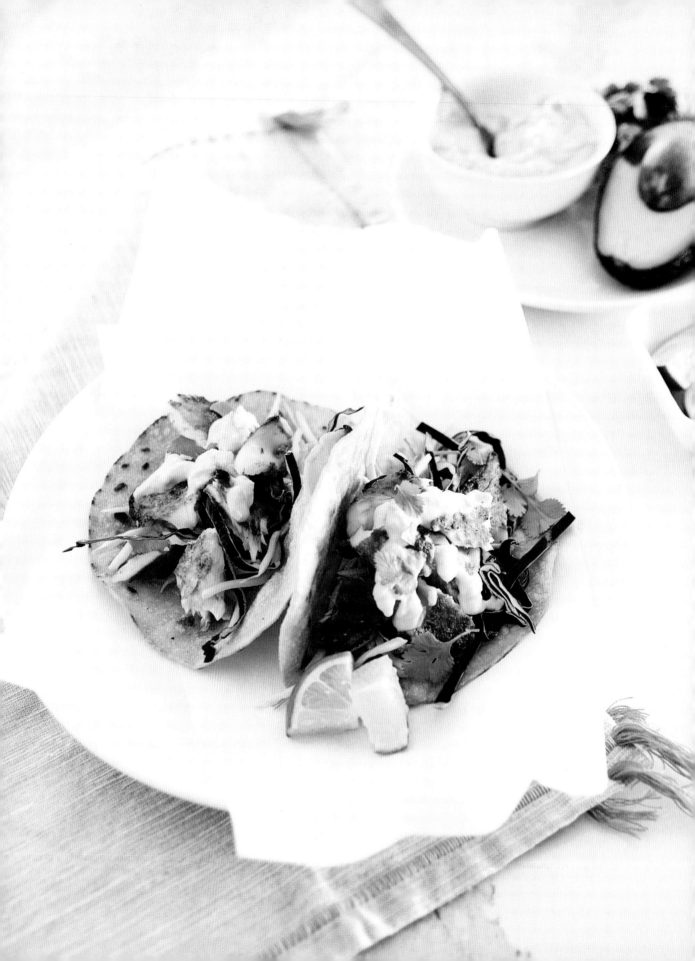

Colorful Fish Tacos

You don't have to wait for Taco Tuesday to make this awesome recipe. It's the perfect way to include healthy fish and added vegetables to your diet. Tilapia is a nice mild fish to start with if fish is a new addition to your diet, but if you're feeling more adventurous, you can use catfish or shrimp with this recipe too.

Yield: 8 tacos or 4 portions (2 tacos per portion)

Prep Time: 30 minutes

Cook Time: 15 minutes

1 tablespoon (15 ml) extra-virgin olive oil

½ teaspoon smoked or regular paprika

½ teaspoon cumin

½ teaspoon chili powder

½ teaspoon onion powder

½ teaspoon garlic powder

½ teaspoon Himalayan pink salt (use more or less to taste)

¼ teaspoon cayenne pepper

¼ cup (60 ml) fresh lime juice

1 pound (454 g) tilapia

8 corn tortillas

1 cup (90 g) shredded purple cabbage, for topping

1 cup (70 g) broccoli slaw, for topping

Chopped fresh cilantro, for topping (optional)

Avocado Aioli (page 135), for topping

Lime wedges, for serving

1. In a small bowl, whisk together the olive oil, paprika, cumin, chili powder, onion powder, garlic powder, salt, cayenne, and lime juice. Pour the mixture into a large resealable plastic bag.

2. Add the tilapia to the resealable bag with the mixture, securely seal the bag, and squeeze and shake the bag to coat the fish with the spices. Let the fish marinate in the refrigerator for at least 10 minutes and up to 1 hour.

3. Preheat the oven to 375°F (190°C). Line a large baking sheet with aluminum foil.

4. Place the marinated fish, with the marinade from the bag, onto the prepared baking sheet and bake for 10 minutes, or until the tilapia is fully cooked and easily flakes with a fork. If you would like to add a golden color to the fish, set it under the broiler for 3 to 4 minutes, until slightly brown.

5. Remove the pan from the oven and use a fork to break up the fish into bite-size chunks. Set aside.

6. Equally divide the fish into 4 containers, storing the tortillas, any toppings, and lime wedges in separate containers and/or resealable plastic bags. Store in the refrigerator for up to 4 days. When you are ready to enjoy the tacos, microwave the fish for 30 to 45 seconds and warm the tortillas in a large skillet over high heat. Top with the cabbage, slaw, and cilantro (if using), and serve with the lime wedges and avocado aioli.

Classic and Lean Chili

My dad made a mean chili. When the craving hit at the beginning of fall (like clockwork), he would assemble all his "secret" ingredients and get started on the half-day-long process. It was the only time he would kick us girls out of the kitchen, and we were happy to scram knowing we'd be feasting on his big pot of savory chili for days. This is the "healthified" version I use in my weekly meal preps.

Yield: 6 to 8 portions
Prep Time: 20 minutes
Cook Time: 35 minutes

1 tablespoon (15 ml) extra-virgin olive oil

1 small yellow onion, diced

2 or 3 garlic cloves, minced

1 pound (454 g) lean ground turkey

1 small poblano pepper, seeded and diced (optional)

2 cups (300 g) diced bell pepper

1 cup (120 g) diced carrot

1 cup (30 g) baby spinach

1 can (28 ounces, or 794 g) crushed tomatoes

1 can (15 ounces, or 425 g) black beans, drained and rinsed

1 can (15 ounces, or 425 g) kidney beans, drained and rinsed

1½ tablespoons (22 ml) chili powder

1 teaspoon cumin

1 teaspoon hot sauce

½ teaspoon sea salt

½ teaspoon freshly ground black pepper

1. Heat the olive oil in a large pot with a lid over medium heat for 1 to 2 minutes.

2. Add the onion and garlic, and cook and stir for 2 to 3 minutes. Add the ground turkey, stirring occasionally, until browned, about 10 minutes. Add the remaining ingredients to the pot and stir to combine.

3. Increase the heat to medium-high and bring to a boil. Reduce the heat to medium-low and simmer, covered, for at least 20 minutes and up to 45 minutes, stirring occasionally. Taste the chili as it simmers to add additional spices if needed.

4. Equally divide the chili into 6 to 8 containers. Store in the refrigerator for up to 5 days or freeze up to 3 months. To reheat, warm the chili in a pot over medium heat, stirring occasionally, for 5 to 6 minutes. If using the microwave, place the desired amount in a microwave-safe bowl, loosely cover, and heat for 2 to 3 minutes, stirring halfway through the cooking time.

PRO PREP TIP

This recipe is super flexible! You can use any vegetables and/or beans you have on hand and adjust the spices to your personal taste.

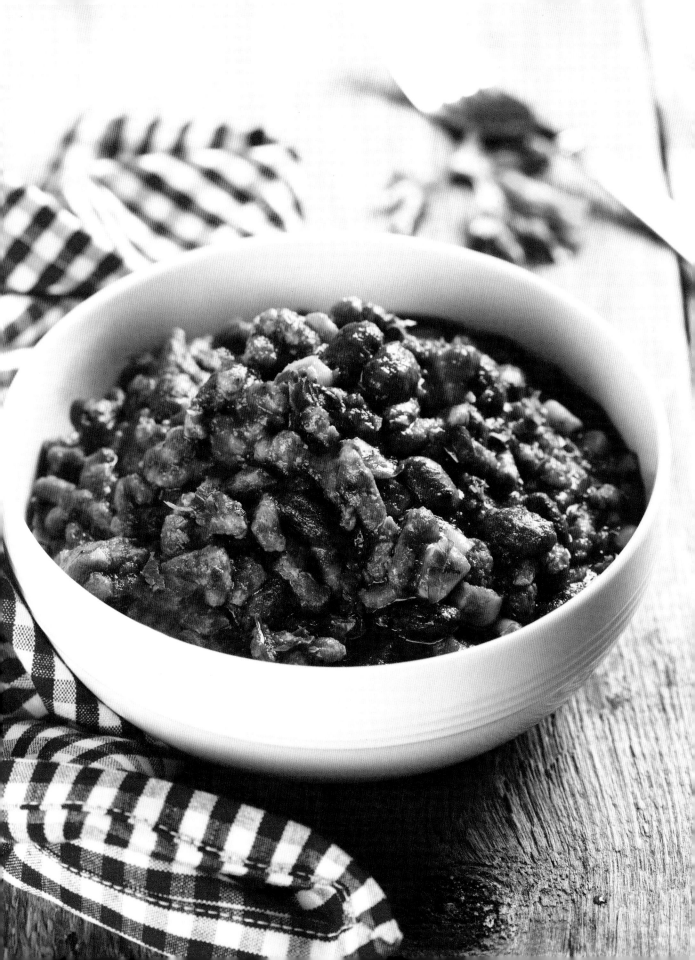

Roasted Vegetables and Chicken Wraps

Yield: 4 portions

Prep Time: 15 minutes

Cook Time: 45 minutes

Roasted vegetables are already tasty, and when they are combined with goat cheese, like in this recipe, they're irresistible.

ROASTED VEGETABLES

1 medium sweet potato, unpeeled and sliced into long strips

1 cup (150 g) cubed squash (frozen or fresh)

3 tablespoons (45 ml) olive oil

¼ cup (60 ml) balsamic vinegar

½ teaspoon dried thyme

½ teaspoon garlic salt

½ teaspoon freshly ground black pepper

1 large onion, thinly sliced

1 large red bell pepper, thinly sliced

CHICKEN

1 tablespoon (15 ml) olive oil

2 large boneless and skinless chicken breasts, sliced in half lengthwise

WRAPS

4 large (10 inches, or 25 cm, each) whole wheat tortillas

4 teaspoons (50 g) Hummus (page 136)

4 teaspoons (13 g) goat cheese (substitute feta or smoked Gouda)

1. **To make the roasted vegetables:** Preheat the oven to 375°F (190°C). Line 2 large, rimmed baking sheets with parchment paper and set aside.

2. In a large bowl, toss together the sweet potato, squash, olive oil, vinegar, thyme, garlic salt, and black pepper. Evenly spread the sweet potato–squash mixture onto one of the prepared baking sheets. Don't rinse out the bowl. Roast in the oven for about 45 minutes, until the vegetables soften and begin to brown. Remove from the oven and let rest for 2 to 3 minutes.

3. Place the onion and bell pepper into the sweet potato–squash bowl and toss with the remaining dressing. Spread the mixture onto the remaining prepared baking sheet. Cook for the last 30 minutes of the sweet potato–squash cooking time, until the vegetables soften and begin to brown. Remove from the oven and let rest for 2 to 3 minutes.

4. **To make the chicken:** Heat the olive oil in a large skillet over medium-high heat. Add the chicken to the skillet without overlapping the pieces. Flip each chicken breast over once the underside is golden brown, about 6 minutes per side. To check for doneness, slice through one of the chicken breasts to see that the meat is white and the juices run clear.

5. Remove the chicken from the pan and let cool on a clean cutting board, 6 to 7 minutes. Diagonally slice it into strips.

6. You can begin to assemble the wraps or store the chicken strips in an airtight container in the refrigerator for up to 4 days.

7. **To assemble the wraps:** Lay out the tortillas on a clean surface. Spread about 1 teaspoon of hummus on each tortilla, leaving a ½-inch (13 mm) border around the edges. Top each tortilla with one-quarter each of the roasted vegetable mixtures and sliced chicken and 1 teaspoon of the goat cheese.

8. To roll the wrap, start at the edge closest to you, fold the tortilla up slightly with your thumbs, fold the sides in with your fingers, and continue to tuck and roll to create a burrito-like wrap. Repeat with the remaining tortillas.

9. Place each wrap into a container and store in the refrigerator for up to 2 days. If you are making more than 2 days' worth of wraps, store the toppings separately for up to 5 days and assemble the wraps the day of eating.

PRO PREP TIP

For a protein-packed wrap, substitute the tortilla with this easy and delicious three-ingredient wrap. Here's how to make it:

Nonstick cooking spray (olive, coconut, or avocado oil)

2 cups (450 g) cottage cheese

2 large eggs

1 teaspoon Italian seasoning (or a mixture of ½ teaspoon garlic powder, ½ teaspoon black pepper, and ½ teaspoon oregano)

1. Preheat the oven to 350°F (180°C). Line a small (quarter-size) baking sheet with parchment paper. Spray the parchment paper with olive, coconut, or avocado oil cooking spray.

2. Add the cottage cheese, egg, and seasoning to a food processor or blender and process until smooth. Pour the mixture onto the prepared baking sheet and spread it into a thin layer (but not thin enough to see the parchment paper through it).

3. Bake for 35 to 45 minutes, until the wrap is soft but browned on top. Let cool for 5 minutes, then assemble following steps 7 through 9.

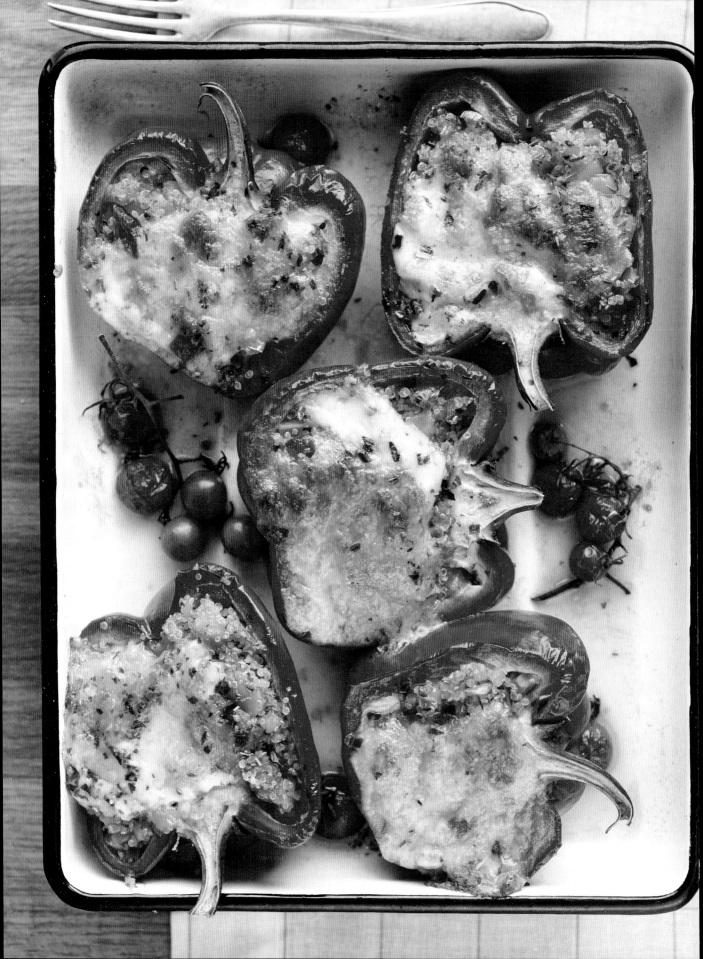

Ground Chicken and Quinoa–Stuffed Peppers

Yield: 4 portions

Prep Time: 20 minutes

Cook Time: 20 minutes

This is one of my favorite recipes for meal prep; it's also a dish I love serving my family and friends for dinner. It's yummy, satisfying, and healthy. I also like that I can play with the ingredients a bit. Depending on your taste (or the tastes of your guests), consider adding some heat to your stuffed peppers with diced jalapeños, smoked paprika, cayenne pepper, or crushed red pepper flakes.

1 tablespoon (15 ml) olive oil

2 garlic cloves, minced

½ large yellow onion, chopped

1 pound (454 g) lean ground chicken

1 cup (180 g) diced tomatoes (canned or fresh)

1 teaspoon garlic powder

1 teaspoon chili powder

1 teaspoon sea salt

1 cup (185 g) cooked quinoa

4 large sweet red bell peppers, tops cut off and seeds removed

¼ cup (30 g) part-skim shredded cheddar cheese (optional)

Low-fat sour cream or plain Greek-style yogurt, for topping (optional)

1. Preheat the oven to 350°F (180°C).

2. Heat the olive oil in a large skillet with a lid over medium-high heat for 30 seconds.

3. Add the garlic and onion, and cook and stir for about 2 minutes. Add the ground chicken. Chop or crumble the meat using a wooden spoon or silicone-coated utensil. Cook the meat for 5 to 8 minutes, stirring frequently to break up the meat.

4. When the meat has browned, add the tomatoes, garlic powder, chili powder, and sea salt to the skillet and cover. Reduce the heat to low and simmer for 5 to 6 minutes, stirring occasionally. Add the quinoa and stir to combine.

5. Place the peppers, cut sides up, in a deep baking dish and bake for approximately 5 minutes, until they begin to soften.

6. Spoon the meat-quinoa mixture into each pepper and fill to the top. Sprinkle with the cheese.

7. Place each stuffed pepper into a container. Store in the refrigerator for up to 4 days. To reheat, warm in the oven at 350°F (180°C) for 5 to 6 minutes or microwave for 1 to 2 minutes. Top with the sour cream (if using).

Mediterranean Chicken

Yield: 8 portions

Prep Time: 15 minutes

Cook Time: 25 minutes

Pair this flavorful chicken dish with Crispy Sweet Potato Medallions (page 125) or Cauliflower Rice (page 124).

3 tablespoons (45 ml) olive oil, divided

4 large boneless and skinless chicken breasts (8 ounces, or 227 g, each), sliced in half lengthwise

4 garlic cloves, smashed

1 medium yellow onion, thinly sliced

2 large lemons, sliced

1 cup (150 g) cherry or grape tomatoes

1 cup (100 g) pitted green olives

¾ cup (180 ml) low-sodium chicken stock

1 teaspoon crushed red pepper flakes (optional)

Himalayan pink salt, to taste

Freshly ground black pepper, to taste

1. Heat 2 tablespoons (30 ml) of the olive oil in a large skillet with a lid over medium-high heat for 30 seconds. Place the chicken fillets into the skillet and cook each side until golden brown, 3 to 4 minutes per side. Reduce the heat to medium and transfer the chicken to a plate.

2. Add the remaining 1 tablespoon (15 ml) olive oil, garlic, and onion to the skillet. Cook over medium heat until the onion is soft but not yet brown, 2 to 3 minutes.

3. Add the lemon slices, tomatoes, olives, and chicken stock to the skillet. Place the chicken breasts back into the pan, on top. Season with the red pepper flakes (if using), pink salt, and black pepper. Reduce the heat to low, cover, and simmer until the chicken is just cooked through, about 15 minutes.

4. Place each fillet, with the cooking liquid, into a container. Store in the refrigerator for up to 4 days. To reheat, warm in a skillet over medium heat until heated through, stirring occasionally.

PRO PREP TIP

To freeze, place 1 or 2 fillets of cooled chicken in a resealable plastic freezer bag with a few tablespoons (45 ml) of cooled cooking liquid. Squeeze out any air and tightly seal the bag. Enjoy within 3 to 4 months. To reheat, empty the contents of the bag into a skillet over medium heat, cover, and warm until heated through, stirring occasionally.

Lemony Pasta Salad with Asparagus

Yield: 4 portions

Prep Time: 10 minutes

Cook Time: 20 minutes

This fresh and easy pasta salad is guaranteed to satisfy you on its own, but I like to add a protein to balance out the dish. The following lean sources of protein are great additions to this recipe: grilled chicken, hard-boiled eggs (page 37), shrimp, or sliced steak.

8 ounces (227 g) whole wheat fusilli or penne pasta

1 pound (454 g) asparagus, trimmed and chopped into bite-size pieces

¼ cup (25 g) grated Parmesan cheese

2 tablespoons (30 ml) extra-virgin olive oil

1 tablespoon (15 ml) fresh lemon juice

1 teaspoon grated lemon zest

½ teaspoon Himalayan pink salt

½ teaspoon freshly ground black pepper

1. Cook the pasta according to the package directions, adding the asparagus during the last 3½ minutes of the cooking time.

2. Transfer a ladleful (about ¾ cup, or 180 ml) of the cooking liquid to a large bowl. Set aside. Drain the pasta and asparagus, and rinse under cold water until cool, 30 to 45 seconds.

3. Transfer the drained pasta and asparagus to the bowl with the reserved pasta water. Add the Parmesan, olive oil, lemon juice and zest, pink salt, and black pepper. Toss to combine.

4. Equally divide the pasta salad into 4 containers. Store in the refrigerator for up to 5 days.

Ginger-Soy Chicken Thighs

Yield: 4 portions

Prep Time: 30 minutes

Cook Time: 35 minutes

Chicken is my go-to protein when it comes to weekly meal prep, but I'll admit that chicken can get a little boring. This is just the recipe you need to shake things up. (I have a feeling I'll be hearing from you about this one!) Searing the thighs before roasting them in the oven helps to hold in moisture and prevent the chicken from becoming soggy.

2¼ pounds (1 kg) boneless and skinless chicken thighs (about 12 chicken thighs)

½ cup (80 g) thinly sliced red onion

2 tablespoons (20 g) minced garlic (you can substitute 1 teaspoon garlic powder)

2 tablespoons (12 g) minced peeled ginger or 1 teaspoon ground ginger

¼ cup (60 ml) low-sodium soy sauce

3 tablespoons (45 ml) balsamic vinegar

2 teaspoons (10 ml) olive oil

Dash cayenne pepper

PRO PREP TIP

To reduce the sodium in any dish that calls for soy sauce, cut it with balsamic vinegar. The sweetness of the balsamic vinegar mellows the salty punch of the soy sauce.

1. Place the chicken thighs into a large resealable plastic bag. Set aside.

2. In a medium bowl, whisk together all the remaining ingredients. Add the marinade to the resealable bag with the chicken, securely seal the bag, and shake to coat the chicken. Let the chicken marinate in the refrigerator for a minimum of 20 minutes and up to 6 hours.

3. When you are ready to cook the chicken, preheat the oven to 400°F (200°C). Heat a large skillet over medium-high heat. Using tongs, remove the thighs from the plastic bag and place into the skillet, reserving the marinade in the plastic bag. Cook the chicken thighs until browned, 2 to 3 minutes per side, and remove from the heat. Transfer the seared chicken to a baking dish with a lid and pour the reserved marinade from the bag onto the chicken.

4. Bake for 30 minutes, until the chicken is cooked through. To check the chicken for doneness, slice one of the chicken thighs in half. The inside should be fully cooked; if you see a lot of pink, bake it for 5 more minutes. For a more accurate reading, use a meat thermometer to make sure the thighs have reached 165°F (75°C).

5. Equally divide the chicken thighs into 4 containers. Store in the refrigerator for up to 5 days. To reheat, microwave for 2 to 3 minutes.

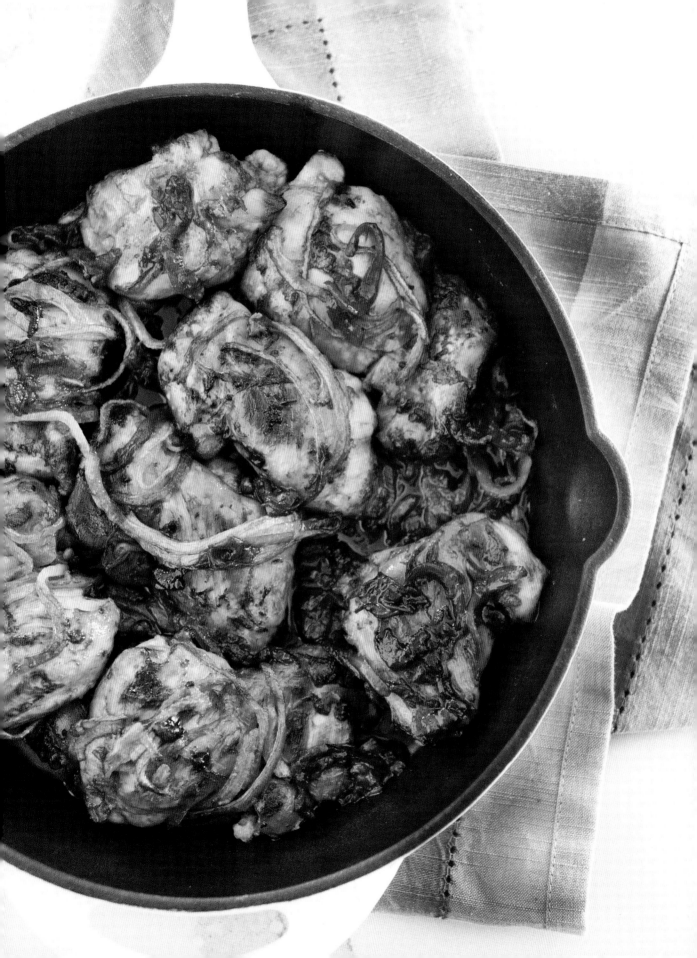

Tomato, Egg, and Lentil Bowls

Yield: 4 portions

Prep Time: 10 minutes

This nutritious bowl will keep you feeling full until your next meal, and it takes mere minutes to prepare (especially if you have the hard-boiled eggs on hand). It's the perfect summer salad that tastes even better after a couple days, as the flavors meld together even more.

1 can (15 ounces, or 425 g) lentils, drained and rinsed

2 medium Roma tomatoes, diced

½ cup (55 g) shredded carrot

2 small scallions, diced

¼ cup (15 g) chopped fresh parsley

3 tablespoons (45 ml) fresh lime juice

3 tablespoons (45 ml) extra-virgin olive oil

Himalayan pink salt, to taste

Freshly ground black pepper, to taste

Hot sauce (I like Frank's RedHot Original sauce), to taste

4 Hard-Boiled Eggs in the Oven (page 37), peeled and sliced

1. Place the lentils, tomatoes, carrot, scallions, and parsley into a large bowl.

2. Drizzle the lime juice and olive oil over the lentil-tomato mixture and stir to combine. Stir in the pink salt, black pepper, and hot sauce.

3. Equally divide the mixture into 4 portions and top each portion with a sliced hard-boiled egg. Store in the refrigerator for up to 5 days.

Roasted Butternut Squash Soup

Yield: 4 or 5 portions

Prep Time: 15 minutes

Cook Time: 50 minutes

This soup will warm you up and give you a good dose of micronutrients (vitamins and minerals). It will also taste as though it took hours to make, but it's super simple and quick to prepare. To make this soup into a heartier meal, consider adding shredded chicken, Crispy Cubed Tofu (page 120), or quinoa to your bowl of goodness.

1 large butternut squash (or 3 cups, or 450 g, frozen cubed butternut squash)

1 tablespoon (15 ml) extra-virgin olive oil

¼ cup (40 g) diced yellow onion

2 garlic cloves, minced

2½ cups (600 ml) low-sodium vegetable broth

¼ cup (60 ml) unsweetened coconut milk (from a carton) or almond milk

Sea salt, to taste

Freshly ground black pepper, to taste

Curry powder, to taste (optional)

Cayenne pepper, to taste (optional)

1. Preheat the oven to 400°F (200°C) and line a large baking sheet with aluminum foil.

2. Cut the butternut squash in half lengthwise and pierce a few times with a fork. Place the squash halves on the baking sheet, flesh sides down. Bake until tender when pierced with a fork, 25 to 30 minutes. (If using frozen cubed squash, bake for 15 minutes.)

3. Remove from the oven, let cool, and carefully scoop out the flesh of the squash into a large bowl. Set aside.

4. Warm the olive oil in a large pot with a lid over medium heat until shimmering, 30 to 60 seconds. Add the onion and garlic, and cook and stir until soft and aromatic, 2 to 3 minutes. Add the broth and roasted squash, and stir to combine. Increase the heat to medium-high and bring to a boil, then swiftly reduce the heat to medium-low, cover, and simmer for 20 minutes, stirring occasionally.

5. Remove from the heat and let stand for 2 to 3 minutes. Using an immersion blender in a circular motion, blend the soup until smooth, about 1 minute. Slowly add the coconut milk until the desired consistency is achieved and blend once again to combine. Season to taste with the sea salt, black pepper, curry powder (if using), and cayenne pepper (if using).

6. Equally divide into 4 or 5 containers. Store in the refrigerator for up to 6 days. To reheat, microwave for 2 minutes or warm in pot over medium heat for 4 to 5 minutes, stirring frequently.

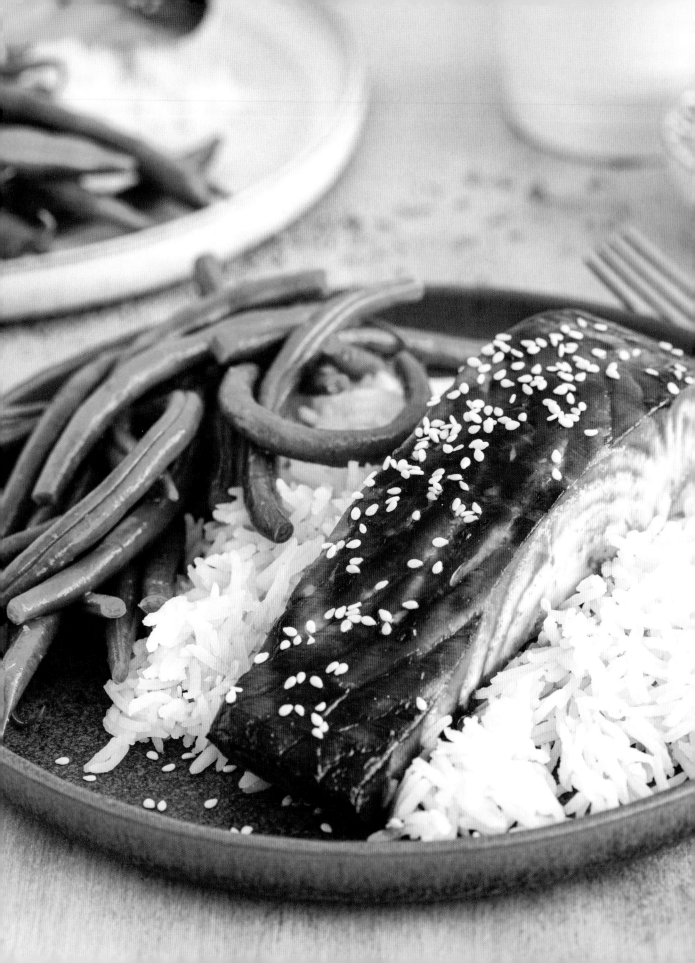

Pan-Fried Teriyaki Salmon

Yield: 4 portions

Prep Time: 30 minutes

Cook Time: 10 minutes

You're likely to find a few different options when buying salmon at your local grocery store or market: fresh or frozen, wild or farmed, whole fish or individual fillets. What you purchase is a matter of preference and/or availability in most cases; however, if you are buying a whole side, you'll want to cut the piece into equal-size portions before cooking. I love this tangy salmon served on top of Cauliflower Rice (page 124).

2 tablespoons (30 ml) olive oil

4 skinless salmon fillets (each 6 ounces, or 170 g)

1 small white onion, sliced

3 garlic cloves, halved and thinly sliced

¼ cup (60 ml) teriyaki sauce

Sesame seeds, for topping (optional)

1. Preheat the oven to 375°F (190°C).

2. Heat the olive oil in a large skillet over medium heat for 1 minute. Place the salmon fillets in the skillet without overcrowding. Place the sliced onions, garlic, and teriyaki sauce on top of the fillets.

3. Cook for 3 to 4 minutes on each side, or until the salmon is fully cooked and easily flakes with a fork. Sprinkle with sesame seeds (if using).

4. Place each fillet into a container with the cooking liquid. Store in the refrigerator for up to 4 days. To reheat, place the fish on a baking sheet and warm in an oven at 400°F (200°C) for 3 to 4 minutes. You can also microwave for 1 minute per fillet, though oven reheating is preferred for this dish.

Turkey and Kale Soup with Super Grains

Yield: 6 to 8 portions

Prep Time: 15 minutes

Cook Time: 45 minutes

This savory soup doesn't require you to roast a turkey in order to prepare it; however, making this recipe around the holidays is a great way to repurpose leftover turkey. Feel free to swap out the pearled spelt and barley with a whole grain of your choice (e.g., brown rice, quinoa, farro, or wheat berries).

32 ounces (4 cups, or 946 ml) chicken stock

2 cups (475 ml) cold water

½ cup (100 g) pearled spelt, rinsed

½ cup (100 g) barley, rinsed

1 tablespoon (15 ml) extra-virgin olive oil

1 medium yellow onion, diced

3 large garlic cloves, minced

1 cup (110 g) cooked crumbled turkey kielbasa

1 cup (140 g) cooked cubed roast turkey (buy precooked turkey and cut into cubes; look for low-sodium and nitratefree brands)

1 to 2 cups (180 to 360 g) diced tomatoes (canned or fresh)

2 cups (134 g) chopped kale

½ teaspoon sea salt

½ teaspoon freshly ground black pepper

½ teaspoon dried oregano

½ teaspoon crushed red pepper flakes

1. Bring the chicken stock and cold water to a boil in a large pot with a lid over medium-high heat.

2. Once boiling, add the spelt and barley, reduce the heat to low, and simmer for 35 to 40 minutes.

3. Meanwhile, heat the olive oil in a large skillet over medium heat for 1 to 2 minutes. Add the onion and garlic to the skillet, and cook and stir for 2 more minutes. Add the turkey kielbasa and roast turkey to the skillet and toss to heat through, 4 to 5 minutes.

4. Remove the skillet from the heat and transfer the contents to the pot with the stock and grains.

5. Add the tomatoes, kale, sea salt, black pepper, oregano, and red pepper flakes, and simmer, covered, for 10 to 15 minutes.

6. Equally divide into 6 to 8 containers. Store in the refrigerator for up to 5 days or freeze for up to 6 months. To reheat, warm in a pot over medium-high heat for 7 to 8 minutes or microwave each portion for 1½ to 2 minutes.

Mixed Bean Salad

This recipe has been a repeat in my meal-prep plan for years now. It's quick and easy, and tastes even better on days two and three. Feel free to change up the types of beans depending on what you have on hand.

Yield: 4 portions

Prep Time: 10 minutes

DRESSING

¼ cup (60 ml) avocado oil

¼ cup (60 ml) red wine vinegar

½ teaspoon dried oregano

½ teaspoon freshly ground black pepper

½ teaspoon sea salt

SALAD

1 cup (250 g) canned chickpeas, drained and rinsed

1 cup (250 g) canned black beans, drained and rinsed

1 cup (200 g) edamame, shelled (thawed if using frozen)

1 cup (120 g) chopped cucumber

1 cup (150 g) halved cherry tomatoes

1 cup (150 g) diced orange bell pepper

1. **To make the dressing:** Place all the dressing ingredients into a Mason jar or sealable container and secure with the lid. Shake to combine. Set aside.

2. **To make the salad:** In a large salad bowl, combine all the salad ingredients. Pour the dressing over the salad and toss to coat.

3. Evenly divide the salad into 4 containers. Store in the refrigerator for up to 5 days, tossing the salad each day to mix it up and refresh it.

Chicken Tortilla Soup

Yield: 6 to 8 portions

Prep Time: 20 minutes

Cook Time: 50 minutes

I promise this soup will soothe and warm your soul. I hope you enjoy this one as much as I do.

3 boneless and skinless chicken breasts (each 4 to 6 ounces, or 113 to 170 g)

1 tablespoon (15 ml) olive oil

1 medium white onion, chopped

3 garlic cloves, minced

2 teaspoons chili powder

1 teaspoon dried oregano

1 large red bell pepper, diced

1 can (28 ounces, or 794 g) diced tomatoes

3 cups (700 ml) low-sodium chicken broth

1 cup (240 ml) water

1 cup (150 g) whole corn kernels (optional)

1 can (15 ounces, or 425 g) black beans, rinsed and drained

¼ cup (4 g) chopped fresh cilantro (optional)

1 cup (240 g) Guacamole (page 133), for topping (optional)

1 cup (240 g) low-fat sour cream, for topping (optional)

2 scallions, chopped, for topping (optional)

1 recipe Baked Tortilla Triangles (page 128), for serving (optional)

1. Place the chicken breasts into a large saucepan with a lid. Add enough water to just cover the chicken. Cover the pot and bring to a boil over medium-high heat. Reduce the heat to medium-low and simmer the chicken until the meat is no longer pink, about 12 minutes.

2. Transfer the chicken breasts to a large bowl, and using 2 forks, shred the chicken meat. Set aside.

3. Heat the olive oil in a large pot with a lid over medium heat. Add the onion and garlic, and cook and stir until both are soft, 2 to 3 minutes.

4. Add the chili powder, oregano, bell pepper, tomatoes, broth, and water. Bring to a boil, then reduce the heat to low and simmer for 5 to 10 minutes partially covered.

5. Add the shredded chicken, corn (if using), beans, and cilantro (if using). Cook for 10 more minutes, covered, stirring once or twice. Remove from the heat.

6. Equally divide the soup into 6 to 8 containers, storing any toppings and the tortilla triangles (if using) in separate containers. Store in the refrigerator for up to 6 days. To reheat, warm in a pot over medium-high heat for 4 to 5 minutes, stirring frequently, or microwave for 1½ to 2 minutes. Top with the guacamole (if using), sour cream (if using), and scallions (if using). Serve with the baked tortilla wedges (if using).

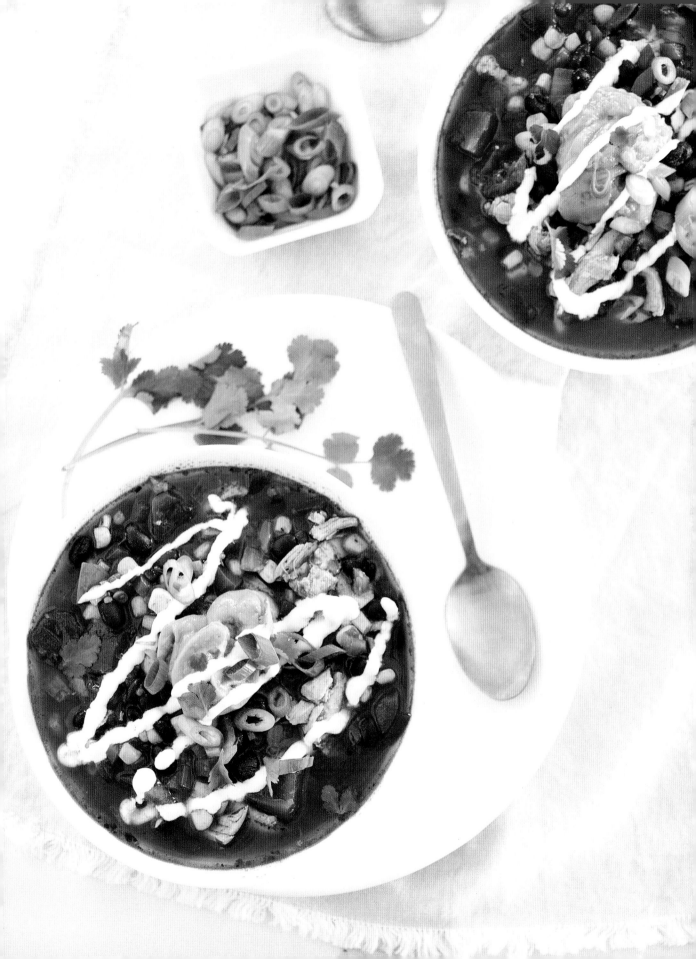

Savory Rice and Beans

Yield: 4 to 6 portions

Prep Time: 20 minutes

Cook Time: 20 minutes

The pairing of rice and beans can be found in cuisines all over the world. The combination creates a complete protein, which makes this recipe an excellent choice for vegetarians and meat eaters alike.

2 cans (15 ounces, or 425 g, each) black or white beans, rinsed and drained

1 teaspoon olive oil

1 medium onion of choice, chopped

1 large red bell pepper, chopped

1½ cups (350 ml) vegetable broth

1 cup (190 g) quick-cooking or instant brown rice

1 teaspoon chili powder

1 teaspoon ground cumin

1 teaspoon turmeric

½ teaspoon garlic salt

½ teaspoon freshly ground black pepper

3 cups (90 g) baby spinach

½ teaspoon sea salt

½ cup (8 g) chopped fresh cilantro, for topping (optional)

Lime wedges, for serving

1. Place the beans into a medium pot with enough water to just cover them and bring to a boil. Reduce the heat to medium-low and simmer for 20 minutes, stirring occasionally.

2. Meanwhile, heat the olive oil in a large saucepan with a lid over medium heat for 30 seconds. Add the onion and bell pepper, and cook and stir for 4 to 5 minutes. Pour the broth into the skillet and bring to a boil (you may need to slightly increase the heat). Once the broth is boiling, add the rice and reduce the heat to low. Cover and simmer for 5 to 6 minutes, until the rice is cooked.

3. When the rice is cooked, add the chili powder, cumin, turmeric, garlic salt, and black pepper. Stir well to combine. Add the beans and spinach, and cook, covered, for 5 to 6 more minutes. If there is a lot of liquid in the skillet, leave the lid off and cook until mostly evaporated. Remove from the heat, season with the sea salt, and let cool slightly.

4. Equally divide the rice and beans into 4 to 6 containers. Top with the cilantro (if using) and store in the refrigerator for up to 5 days. When ready to enjoy, microwave for 1 to 2 minutes and serve with the lime wedges.

"Not Your Mama's Meatloaf" Muffins

Yield: 12 muffins or 4 portions (3 muffins per portion)

Prep Time: 15 minutes

Cook Time: 40 minutes

These protein-packed muffins are perfectly portioned for meal prep. It is one of those classic recipes where the cooking method and ingredients can be tweaked to your personal preference or what you have on hand in your kitchen (see Pro Prep Tips below).

Nonstick cooking spray (olive or avocado oil)

2 pounds (907 g) lean ground turkey

3 egg whites

1 cup (80 g) whole wheat bread crumbs or quick-cooking oats

½ teaspoon ground cumin

½ teaspoon dried thyme

2 teaspoons dry mustard

2 teaspoons freshly ground black pepper

2 teaspoons chipotle pepper spice

1 teaspoon Himalayan pink salt

2 teaspoons garlic powder

1 small yellow onion, diced

2 large celery ribs, diced

¼ cup (60 g) tomato paste

½ cup (120 ml) barbecue sauce (optional)

1. Preheat the oven to 375°F (190°C). Spray a 12-cup muffin tin or two 6-cup muffin tins with the nonstick cooking spray. Set aside.

2. To a large bowl, add all the ingredients, except the barbecue sauce, and combine well. Scoop the mixture out of the bowl using a large spoon or ice-cream scoop and fill each muffin tin.

3. Bake for 40 minutes, or until cooked through (no longer pink inside or a meat thermometer reaches 165°F, or 75°C). At the 30-minute mark, take the pan out of the oven and brush each muffin with the barbecue sauce (if using), then continue cooking.

4. Place 3 meatloaf muffins each in 4 containers. Store in the refrigerator for up to 5 days. To reheat, microwave for about 1 minute.

PRO PREP TIPS

* This recipe calls for lean ground turkey, but you can substitute any lean meat and end up with the same delicious result.

* Turn this into a loaf by baking the mixture in a loaf pan instead of a muffin tin. Increase the cooking time to 1 hour.

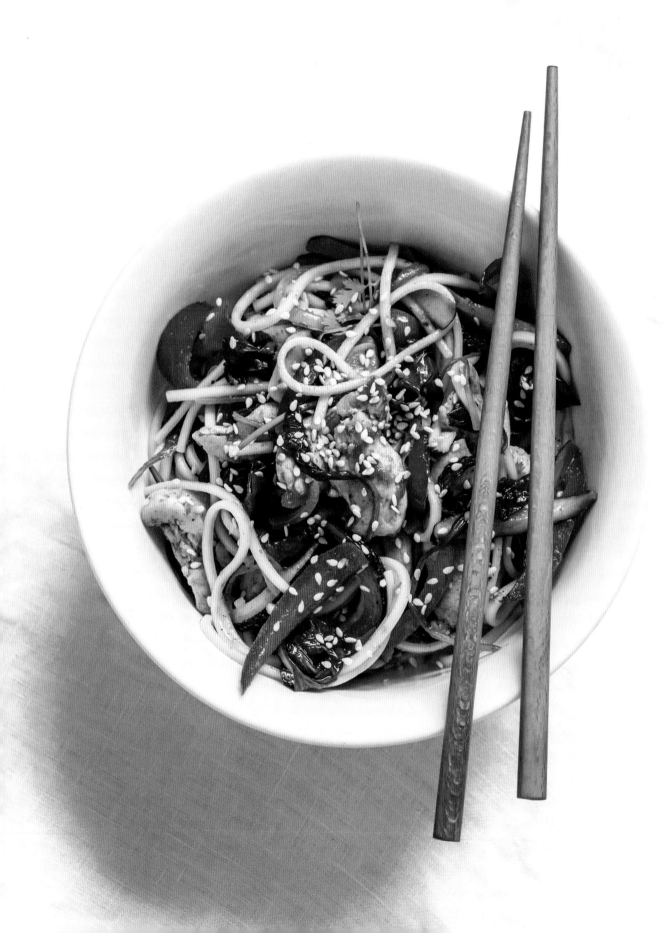

Soba Noodle Stir-Fry

This is the perfect weeknight dinner! If you like your food spicy like I do, add some heat to this dish before serving with 1 to 2 teaspoons of sriracha per portion.

Yield: 4 portions

Prep Time: 20 minutes

Cook Time: 10 minutes

SAUCE

1 teaspoon minced garlic

½ teaspoon minced ginger

½ cup (120 ml) tamari

¼ cup (60 ml) sesame oil

STIR-FRY

1 teaspoon sesame oil

1 cup (92 g) sliced bell pepper

1 cup (110 g) shredded carrot

1 cup (113 g) sliced zucchini

1 cup (70 g) sliced mushrooms

1 cup (90 g) chopped broccoli

½ cup (58 g) sliced red onion

2 cups (60 g) chopped spinach

2 cups (228 g) cooked soba noodles (cooked al dente per package instructions, drained, and rinsed with cold water)

1 cup (104 g) sliced cucumber

1 tablespoon (8 g) hemp hearts (optional)

4 boneless and skinless chicken breasts (each 3 to 4 ounces, or 85 to 113 g), sliced

1. **To make the sauce:** In a small bowl, whisk together all the sauce ingredients. Set aside.

2. **To make the stir-fry:** Heat the sesame oil in a large skillet with a lid over medium-high heat. Once the oil is shimmering, add the bell pepper, carrot, zucchini, mushrooms, broccoli, and onion. Cook, covered, for 4 to 5 minutes, stirring occasionally.

3. Add the spinach and toss for another minute, until the spinach is slightly wilted and incorporated into the vegetable mix. Add the sauce and noodles to the pan. Use silicone-handle tongs to toss the noodles and coat the vegetables in the sauce. Allow the sauce to bubble up and thicken for 1 minute.

4. Equally divide the stir-fry and cucumber slices into 4 containers. Top with the hemp hearts (if using). Do not rinse the skillet.

5. In the same skillet over medium-high heat, cook the sliced chicken. Turn it over when the underside is golden brown, 2 to 3 minutes per side. To check for doneness, cut a slice in half to see that the meat is white and the juices run clear.

6. Equally divide the chicken slices among the containers. Store in the refrigerator for up to 5 days. To reheat, microwave for 1 to 2 minutes per portion or warm in a skillet over medium heat for 4 to 5 minutes, tossing frequently.

PRO PREP TIP

To measure dry noodles, place a bunch of noodles between your thumb and forefinger (like the OK sign) with the tip of your pointer finger at the mid-thumb knuckle. This will measure approximately 4 ounces (227 g) of dry pasta (approximately 2 cups of cooked noodles).

Spanish Rice

When I was growing up, Spanish rice was a family favorite. This dish was actually the first "real" dinner my mom taught me to make. The original recipe calls for ground beef, but it is just as tasty with leaner meats such as ground chicken or turkey. This hearty meal only takes about 30 minutes to prepare from start to finish. I hope your family enjoys it as much as we do.

Yield: 4 to 6 portions

Prep Time: 10 minutes

Cook Time: 20 minutes

1 teaspoon olive oil

1 pound (454 g) lean ground chicken

2 cups (240 g) chopped celery

1 can (28 ounces, or 794 g) diced tomatoes

½ cup (95 g) quick-cooking brown rice

¼ cup (40 g) diced white onion

1 teaspoon chili powder

1 teaspoon garlic powder

Dash Himalayan pink salt

Dash cayenne pepper

½ cup (120 ml) water

1. Heat the olive oil in a large skillet with a lid over medium heat for 30 seconds. Add the ground chicken to the skillet and cook until browned, 8 to 9 minutes.

2. Add the remaining ingredients to the skillet and stir together. Reduce the heat to medium-low, cover, and simmer for 15 minutes, stirring occasionally. Taste the dish to determine whether more seasonings are needed and season accordingly. Remove from the heat and let cool.

3. Equally divide the Spanish rice into 4 to 6 containers. Store in the refrigerator for up to 5 days. To reheat, warm in a skillet over medium heat for 5 to 6 minutes, stirring occasionally, or microwave for 2 to 2½ minutes.

Southwestern Salad

This flavorful and colorful dish is perfect the way it is, but if you would like to add some meat to this plant-based salad, pulled pork or chicken is a great addition.

Yield: 4 portions

Prep Time: 15 minutes

DRESSING

1 large ripe avocado, peeled, pitted, and chopped

½ cup (120 g) plain Greek-style yogurt

2 tablespoons (30 ml) taco seasoning

1 tablespoon (15 ml) ranch seasoning

1 to 4 tablespoons (15 to 60 ml) milk

SALAD

1 cup (230 g) cooked wild rice and bulgur blend (see Pro Prep Tip, below)

1 cup (120 g) corn kernels, fresh or canned

1 cup (250 g) canned black beans, drained and rinsed

¾ cup (135 g) chopped tomato

¾ cup (110 g) diced bell pepper (any color)

¼ cup (50 g) chopped scallion

1 to 2 tablespoons (10 to 20 g) minced garlic

1. **To make the dressing:** Place the avocado, yogurt, taco seasoning, and ranch seasoning in a blender and blend on medium-high speed for 20 seconds. Add the milk, 1 tablespoon (15 ml) at a time, and blend until smooth and the desired consistency is reached. Set aside.

2. **To make the salad:** In a large salad bowl, mix together all the salad ingredients. Pour the dressing over the salad and toss to coat.

3. Equally divide the salad into 4 containers. Store in the refrigerator for up to 5 days, periodically tossing the salad to mix it up and refresh it.

PRO PREP TIP

Most large supermarkets carry some type of grain blend, which is commonly found in the rice aisle. If you can't find a pre-blended mix of wild rice and bulgur, buy them separately and cook according to package directions.

Steak Fajitas

Got 30 minutes? Of course you do! These feisty sheet-pan fajitas will soon be a part of your regular meal-prep routine. This recipe is fast and easy, and the cleanup is a breeze. For a low-carb option, put one serving of steak and vegetable filling into a bowl with 1 cup (30 g) of chopped romaine or baby spinach and add the suggested toppings.

Yield: 8 fajitas or 4 portions (2 fajitas per portion)

Prep Time: 10 minutes

Cook Time: 20 minutes

2 pounds (907 g) flank steak, sliced into ½-inch-thick (13 mm) pieces

1 large red bell pepper, thinly sliced

1 large yellow bell pepper, thinly sliced

1 large green bell pepper, thinly sliced

1 medium red onion, thinly sliced

2 garlic cloves, minced

1 teaspoon ground cumin

½ teaspoon smoked paprika

½ teaspoon chipotle pepper spice (optional)

¼ teaspoon Himalayan pink salt

1½ tablespoons (22 ml) olive oil

3 tablespoons (45 ml) fresh lime juice

8 large (10 inches, or 25 cm, each) whole wheat tortillas (optional; see recipe note, above, for a low-carb option)

2 jalapeños, seeded and thinly sliced, for topping (optional)

Guacamole (store-bought or see recipe on page 133), for topping (optional)

Spicy Greek Yogurt Dip (page 138), for topping (optional)

1. Preheat the oven to 425°F (220°C). Line a large, rimmed baking sheet with aluminum foil. Set aside.

2. Place the sliced steak, bell peppers, and onion into a large resealable plastic bag.

3. In a small bowl, whisk together the garlic, cumin, paprika, chipotle spice (if using), pink salt, olive oil, and lime juice. Pour the mixture into the resealable bag, securely seal the bag, and squeeze and shake the bag to coat the steak and vegetables with the marinade. Let sit for 5 to 10 minutes.

4. Pour the steak and vegetables onto the prepared baking sheet and squeeze any excess marinade on top.

5. Bake for 13 to 15 minutes, stirring halfway through, until the steak reaches desired doneness. Increase the oven setting to broiler and brown the meat and vegetables, 3 to 4 minutes. Watch the meat and vegetables so they don't burn. Remove from the oven and let sit for a few minutes.

6. Equally divide the mixture into 4 containers, storing the tortillas and any toppings in separate containers and/or resealable plastic bags. When you are ready to enjoy, microwave the fajita mixture for 1 to 2 minutes and warm the tortillas in a large skillet over high heat. Assemble the fajitas and top with the jalapeños (if using), guacamole (if using), and yogurt dip (if using).

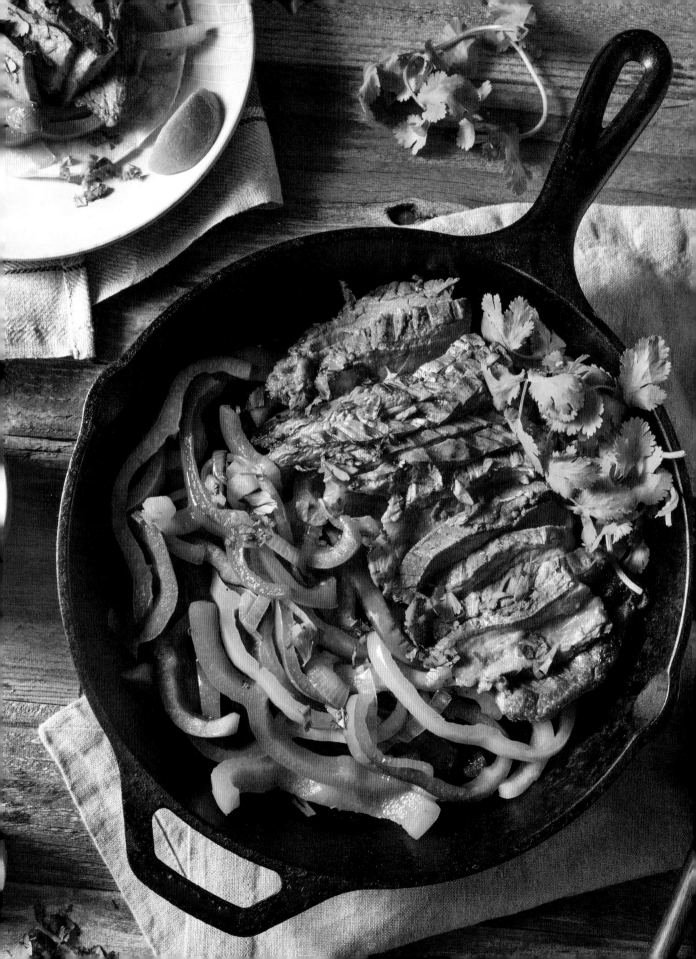

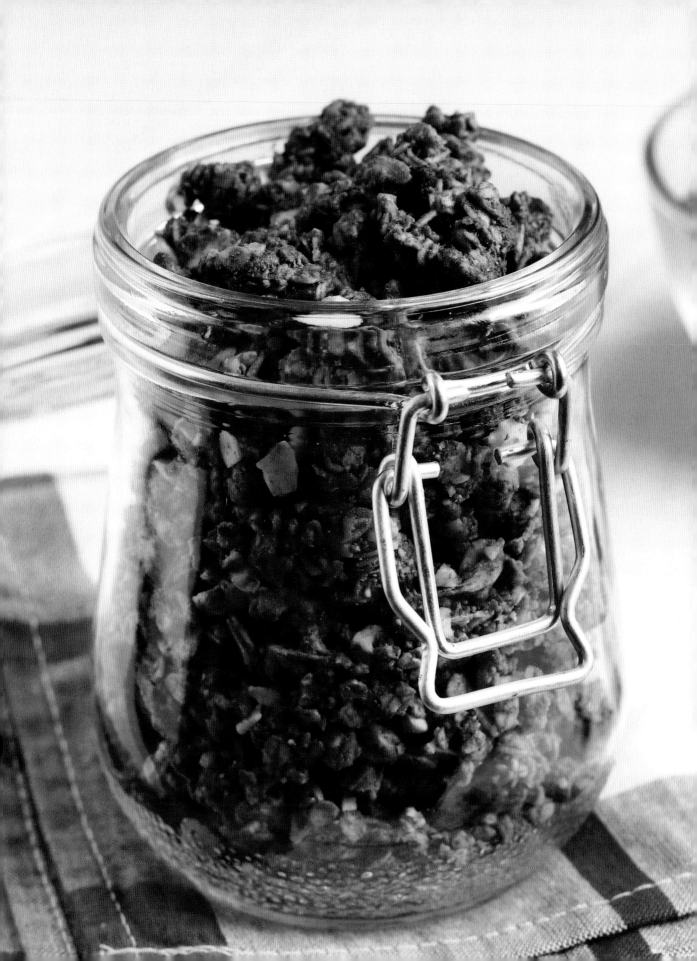

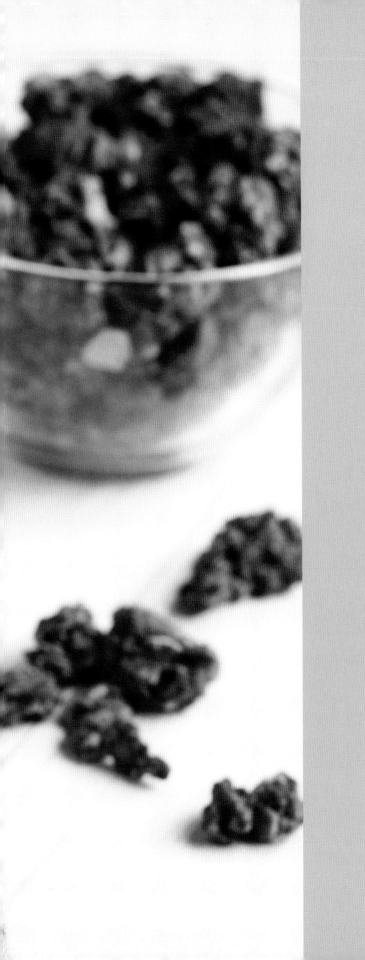

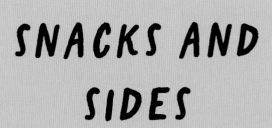

SNACKS AND SIDES

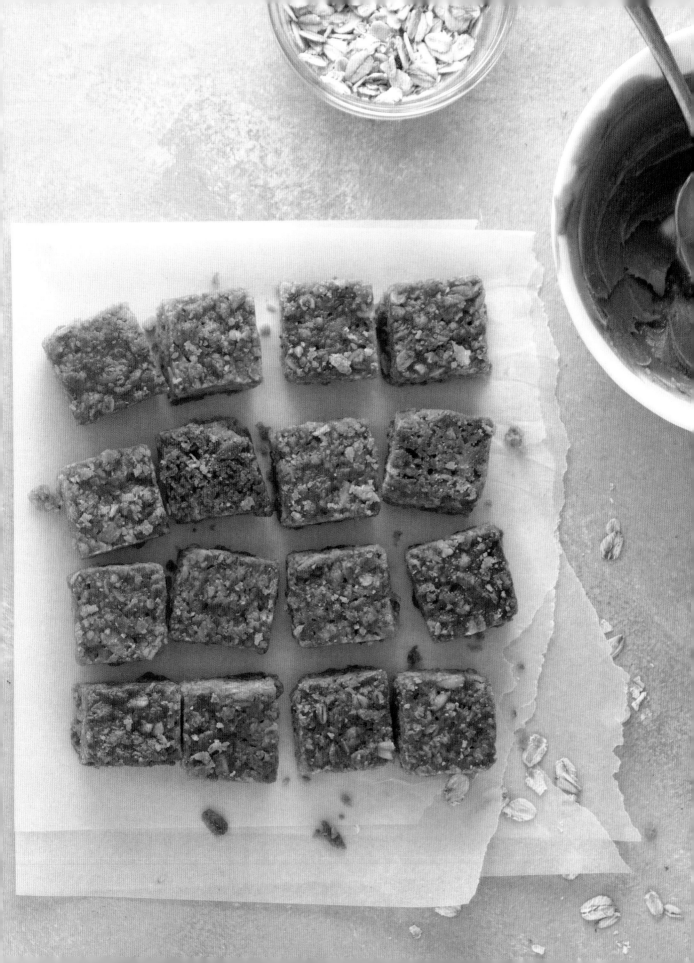

Peanut Butter Brownies

Yield: 16 small squares or 8 medium squares

Prep Time: 15 minutes (plus 15 minutes freezing)

Resisting sweet treats is just not something I want to battle every day. My solution: have sweet yet healthy snacks on hand! You can't beat the simplicity of this recipe, and it's guaranteed to keep your hand out of the cookie jar.

1 cup (260 g) natural peanut butter

½ cup (120 g) coconut oil

½ cup (170 g) raw honey

2 cups (160 g) quick-cooking rolled oats

½ cup (72 g) raw sesame seeds

½ teaspoon salt

½ teaspoon ground cinnamon

½ teaspoon pure vanilla extract

1. Line an 8 × 8-inch (20 × 20 cm) baking pan with parchment paper. Set aside.

2. Melt the peanut butter, coconut oil, and honey in a medium pot over medium heat, stirring frequently, until smooth. Remove from the heat once smooth.

3. Add the oats, sesame seeds, salt, cinnamon, and vanilla to the pot, and stir to combine. Pour the mixture into the prepared pan.

4. Place in the freezer for 15 to 20 minutes, until cool and the brownies start to harden. Remove the brownies from the pan by lifting the parchment paper and place onto a cutting board. Cut into 8 or 16 squares.

5. Place the brownies into containers. Store in the refrigerator for up to 1 week.

Chocolaty Quinoa Squares

Yield: 16 squares

Prep Time: 15 minutes
(plus 2 hours refrigeration)

Cook Time: 30 minutes

If you are looking to make healthier choices but still want to enjoy a sweet treat, this is the recipe for you!

3 cups (555 g) cooked quinoa
(1½ cups, or 192 g, uncooked quinoa)

2½ cups (200 g) rolled oats

¼ cup (28 g) ground flaxseed

¼ cup (16 g) unsalted, shelled pumpkin seeds, ground in a spice or coffee grinder

½ teaspoon Himalayan pink salt

½ teaspoon ground cinnamon

¼ cup (20 g) unsweetened desiccated coconut

⅔ cup (160 ml) almond milk

4 tablespoons (80 g) raw honey

¾ cup (195 g) nut butter of choice

1 tablespoon (14 g) coconut oil

1 bar (3½ ounces, or 100 g) high-quality dark chocolate (75% cacao or higher)

PRO PREP TIP

To freeze these quinoa squares, place a square of parchment or wax paper in between each square and store in a freezer-safe container. Or individually wrap each square in aluminum foil and store in a freezer bag.

1. Preheat the oven to 375°F (190°C). Line a 9 × 9-inch (23 × 23 cm) pan with parchment paper.

2. Combine the quinoa, oats, flaxseed, ground pumpkin seeds, pink salt, cinnamon, coconut, and almond milk in a large bowl.

3. Add the honey, nut butter, and coconut oil to a microwave-safe bowl and microwave in 20-second increments until you can stir and combine them. Add to the bowl with the dry ingredients and stir to combine. Press into the prepared pan.

4. Bake 30 to 35 minutes, until the edges are browned. Remove from the oven and let cool for 15 minutes.

5. To melt the chocolate, break or cut the chocolate into equal-size small pieces. Place it in a clear, microwave-safe glass bowl so you can see it as it melts. Heat for 1 minute. Remove from the microwave and stir (the chocolate will look shiny). Continue to heat in 20-second increments, stirring at each interval, until the chocolate is smooth. Use an offset spatula to spread a layer of melted chocolate onto the cooled quinoa bars.

6. Place the pan in the refrigerator for 2 hours or in the freezer for 30 minutes to set and firm the chocolate. Cut into 16 squares.

7. Place the squares into containers. Store in the refrigerator for up to 6 days or freeze for up to 3 months.

Tropical Energy Balls

Yield: 18 to 20 balls

Prep Time: 20 minutes
(plus 30 minutes refrigeration)

A quick grab-and-go snack that tastes like the warm days of summer? Yes, please! These little morsels make it easy to snack healthy, but I've been known to circle back to these throughout the day and end up with only a couple left. To ensure these will take you through the week, throw 2 or 3 balls in small containers or resealable plastic snack bags as soon as they're prepared and store them in the refrigerator or freezer until they're ready to be eaten.

1 cup (178 g) pitted and halved soft Medjool dates

1 cup (80 g) gluten-free quick-cooking oats

½ cup (85 g) chopped pineapple (fresh or canned and drained)

¼ cup (28 g) flaxseed meal

½ cup (40 g) unsweetened desiccated coconut

1. Add all the ingredients to a food processor or blender and pulse to form a thick paste. Scrape down the sides, if needed, then pulse a couple more times.

2. Scoop out the paste with a tablespoon or a small ice-cream scoop and roll into 18 to 20 balls about the size of a golf ball.

3. Place the balls into containers. Immediately store in the refrigerator for up to 1 week. They are best eaten refrigerated (refrigerated for at least 30 minutes); otherwise, they can be a little soft.

PRO PREP TIP

For these and most other energy/protein ball recipes (see also Amazeballs on page 110 and Energy-Bite Cookies on page 111), if the mixture isn't sticking together as much as you like, try slightly heating the mixture in the microwave, 10 seconds at a time, before rolling into balls.

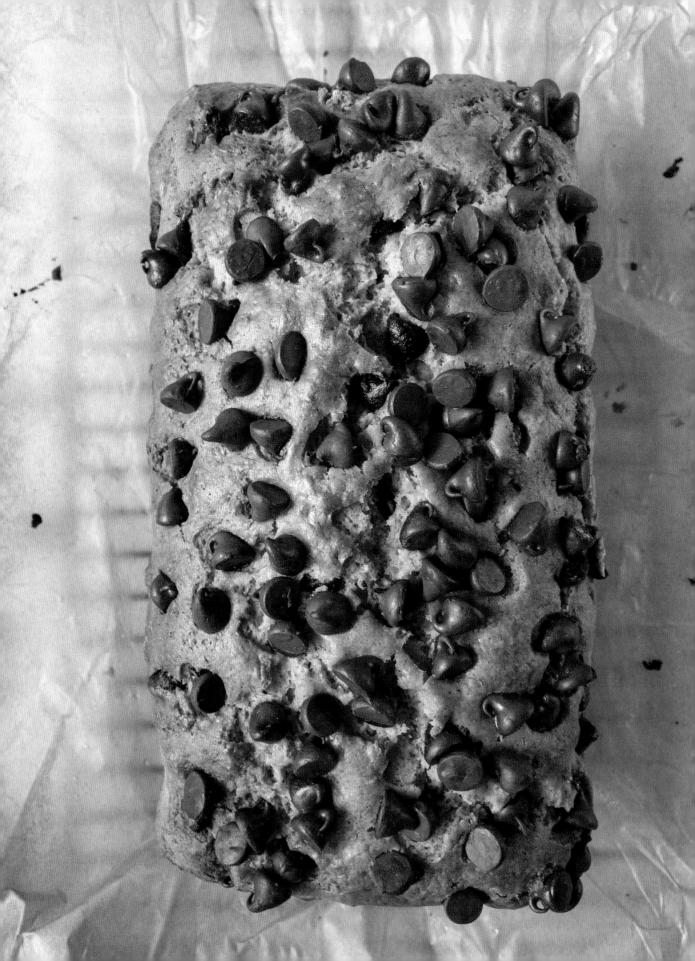

High-Protein Chocolate Chip Banana Bread

Yield: 4 to 6 portions

Prep time: 15 minutes

Cook time: 45 minutes

Ideal for breakfast, a post-workout snack, or a healthy dessert, this banana bread is easy to make and sure to become a favorite in your kitchen.

Nonstick cooking spray (olive or avocado oil) (optional)

1 cup (115 g) almond flour

1 cup (90 g) oat flour

2 scoops vanilla whey protein powder

1 teaspoon baking soda

1 teaspoon baking powder

½ teaspoon Himalayan or sea salt

½ cup (120 g) full-fat plain Greek-style yogurt

⅓ cup (80 ml) pure maple syrup or honey

3 medium bananas, mashed

2 large eggs, at room temperature

1 teaspoon pure vanilla extract

½ cup (85 g) dark chocolate chips, plus more for topping (optional)

1. Preheat the oven to 350°F (180°C). Spray a silicone loaf pan with olive or avocado oil cooking spray (alternatively, line the pan with parchment paper).

2. In a large bowl, stir together the flours, protein powder, baking soda, baking powder, and salt.

3. In a separate large bowl, whisk together the yogurt, maple syrup, mashed bananas, eggs, and vanilla extract.

4. Pour the dry ingredients into the wet ingredients and stir to combine without overmixing. Fold in the chocolate chips.

5. Pour the batter into the prepared loaf pan and smooth out the top with a spatula. Bake for 45 to 55 minutes, until a toothpick inserted into the center comes out mostly clean, checking it at the 30-minute mark; if the loaf seems to be browning too much on top, lightly cover the pan with aluminum foil. Remove from the oven and top with more chocolate chips (if using).

6. Cut the bread into 8 to 12 slices, then place the slices into containers. Store in the refrigerator for up to 1 week.

Apple Cinnamon Walnut Muffins

Yield: 12 muffins

Prep Time: 15 minutes

Cook Time: 30 minutes

These muffins are my favorite on-the-road snack because they are filling but not heavy. Make this recipe your own by substituting a different type of nut. As an alternative to the apples and walnuts, raisins or dried cranberries would be fantastic in these muffins.

Nonstick baking spray (optional)

2 cups (240 g) almond flour

1 cup (80 g) rolled oats

2 teaspoons ground cinnamon, plus more for topping

½ teaspoon salt

1 teaspoon baking soda

½ cup (100 g) coconut sugar

2 large eggs

4 teaspoons (20 g) unsweetened applesauce

1 teaspoon pure vanilla extract

½ cup (120 ml) almond milk

1 large apple of choice, peeled and chopped

½ cup (60 g) chopped walnuts, plus more for topping (optional)

1. Preheat the oven to 350°F (180°C). Line a 12-cup muffin tin or two 6-cup muffin tins with paper liners or spray with baking spray.

2. In a large bowl, combine the almond flour, oats, cinnamon, salt, baking soda, and coconut sugar.

3. In a medium bowl, combine the eggs, applesauce, vanilla, almond milk, apple, and walnuts.

4. Add the wet ingredients to the dry ingredients and gently mix to combine. Scoop the batter into the prepared muffin cups.

5. Bake for 30 minutes, until golden brown and a toothpick inserted into the center of a muffin comes out clean. Remove from the oven and immediately top with the extra walnuts (if using) and a sprinkle of cinnamon.

6. Place the muffins into containers. Store in the refrigerator for up to 1 week.

PRO PREP TIP

To keep the muffins from getting soggy, first let them cool completely on a wire rack, then line an airtight container with a paper towel before storing them. If you are using paper cups to line the muffin tin(s), take off the paper before placing the muffins into the container.

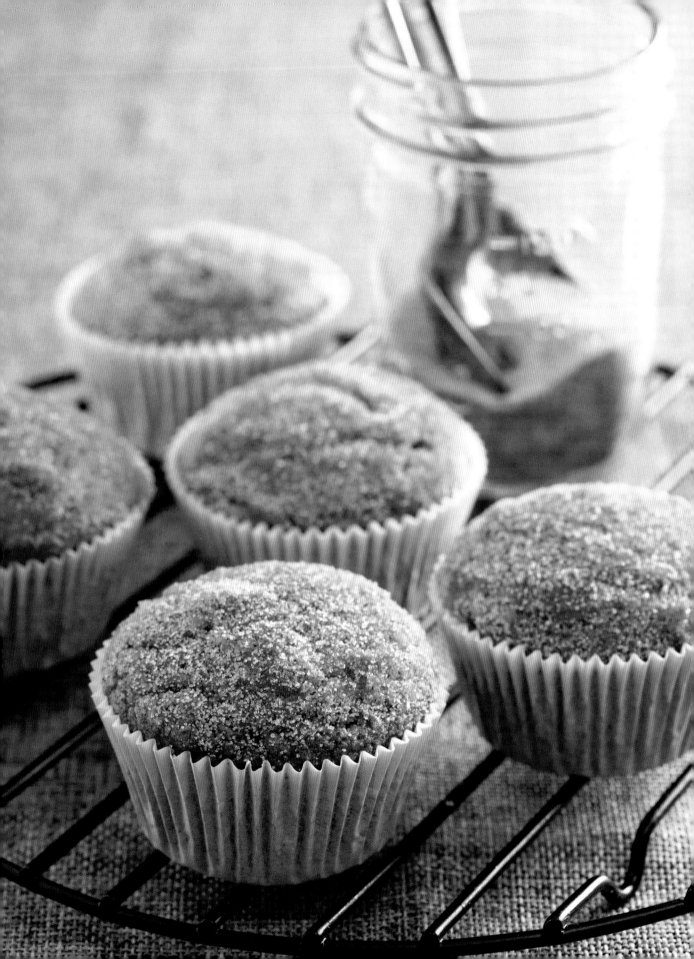

Amazeballs

These family-friendly snacks are a great addition to any healthy eating regimen. Setting aside some time to prepare these balls will be worth it!

Yield: 18 to 25 balls

Prep Time: 20 minutes (plus 30 minutes refrigeration)

16 soft Medjool dates, pitted

¾ cup (82 g) whole raw almonds

½ cup (40 g) unsweetened desiccated coconut

½ teaspoon pure vanilla extract

½ teaspoon Himalayan pink salt

2 tablespoons (22 g) mini dark chocolate or carob chips (optional)

1. Add the dates and almonds to a food processor and pulse until the almonds are coarsely chopped.

2. Add the coconut, vanilla, and pink salt, and pulse until well combined. Test the "batter" to see if it sticks together; if it doesn't, you may need to pulse it a few more times.

3. Transfer the mixture to a large bowl and fold in the chocolate chips (if using). Roll into 18 to 25 balls (a little smaller than a golf ball).

4. Place the balls into containers. Immediately store in the refrigerator for up to 1 week. They are best eaten refrigerated (refrigerated for at least 30 minutes); otherwise, they can be a little soft.

Energy-Bite Cookies

Cookie cravings? I've got you covered with these healthy snacks that are chock-full of guilt-free goodness.

Yield: 24 cookies

Prep Time: 20 minutes

Cook Time: 10 minutes

2 tablespoons (32 g) nut butter of choice

2 tablespoons (28 g) coconut oil

2 cups (160 g) quick-cooking rolled oats

½ cup (40 g) unsweetened desiccated coconut

3 tablespoons (24 g) hemp hearts

1 ripe banana, mashed

1 large egg

⅓ cup (81 g) unsweetened applesauce

½ teaspoon baking soda

½ teaspoon sea salt

½ teaspoon ground cinnamon

½ teaspoon pure vanilla extract

1. Preheat the oven to 325°F (170°C). Line a large baking sheet with parchment paper. Set aside.

2. In separate small bowls, melt the nut butter and coconut oil in the microwave for about 30 seconds.

3. Place all the ingredients into a large bowl (in the order they are listed) and stir with a wooden spoon until well combined.

4. Form 24 balls, each the size of a golf ball, and press them onto the prepared baking sheet to flatten slightly.

5. Bake for 8 to 10 minutes, until the cookies are a light golden brown. Remove from the oven and cool completely in the pan.

6. Place the cookies into containers. Store in the refrigerator for up to 1 week.

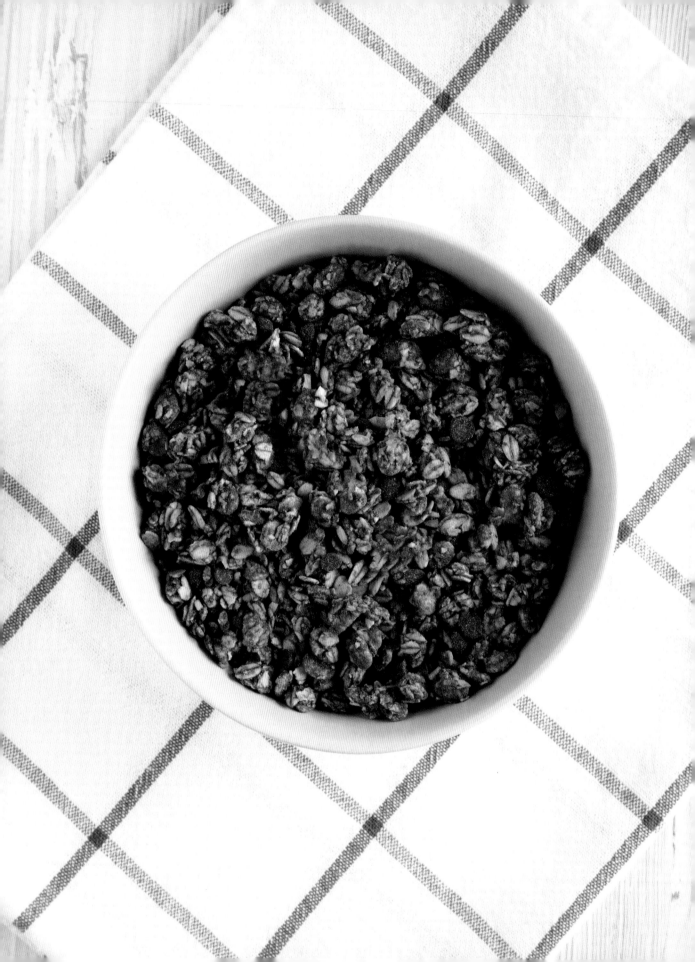

Chocolate Granola

I like to store this granola in 1-pint (16 ounces, or 454 g) Mason jars. This recipe makes 3 Mason jars' worth!

Yield: 3 pounds
(48 ounces, or 1.4 kg)

Prep Time: 15 minutes

Cook Time: 25 minutes

3 cups (240 g) rolled oats

1 cup (80 g) unsweetened desiccated coconut

½ cup (55 g) chopped raw walnuts

½ cup (55 g) chopped raw almonds

½ cup (84 g) chia, flax, or hemp seeds

½ teaspoon Himalayan pink salt

½ cup (60 g) unsweetened cacao or cocoa powder

⅓ cup (80 g) coconut oil

⅓ cup (113 g) raw honey

2 tablespoons (30 ml) extra-virgin olive oil

½ teaspoon pure vanilla extract

1. Preheat the oven to 325°F (170°C). Line a large, rimmed baking sheet with aluminum foil or parchment paper. Set aside.

2. In a large bowl, combine the oats, coconut, walnuts, almonds, seeds, pink salt, and cacao.

3. Place the coconut oil and honey in 2 separate small microwave-safe bowls and heat in the microwave for 20 seconds to melt.

4. Pour the melted coconut oil and honey, along with the olive oil and vanilla, into the bowl with the oats and nuts. Stir to combine until everything is coated. Spread the granola onto the prepared baking sheet.

5. Bake for 15 minutes, then stir and bake for 10 to 15 minutes more. Remove from the oven and cool completely in the pan; the granola will clump and harden as it cools.

6. Equally divide the granola into containers. Store in a cool, dry spot for up to 1 week.

Pumpkin-Spice Granola

Yield: 6 cups (570 g)
Prep Time: 15 minutes
Cook Time: 15 minutes

There are a number of reasons this granola works for meal prep: it's simple to make in big batches, it's half the cost of store-bought granola, it has no refined sugar, and it makes a decadent but healthy snack.

3 cups (240 g) rolled oats

½ cup (55 g) chopped raw almonds

½ cup (55 g) chopped raw pecans

½ cup (75 g) raw sunflower seeds

½ cup (70 g) raw pumpkin seeds

¾ cup (60 g) unsweetened desiccated coconut

1 teaspoon pumpkin spice

½ teaspoon ground cinnamon

½ teaspoon Himalayan pink salt

⅓ cup (80 g) coconut oil

¼ cup (60 ml) pure maple syrup

½ teaspoon almond extract

1. Preheat the oven to 350°F (180°C). Line a large, rimmed baking sheet with aluminum foil or parchment paper. Set aside.

2. In a large bowl, combine the oats, almonds, pecans, sunflower and pumpkin seeds, coconut, pumpkin spice, cinnamon, and pink salt.

3. Melt the coconut oil in a small bowl in the microwave for 15 to 20 seconds. Add the melted coconut oil, maple syrup, and almond extract to the bowl. Stir to combine until everything is coated. Spread the granola onto the prepared baking sheet.

4. Bake the granola for 15 minutes. Watch closely so that the edges don't become too brown. Stir the granola, bringing any browned edges to the inside of the pan. Bake for about 10 more minutes, until the granola is lightly golden brown (check it after 5 minutes). Remove from the oven and cool in the pan, at least 10 minutes; the granola will clump and harden as it cools.

5. Equally divide the granola into containers. Store in a cool, dry spot for up to 1 week or refrigerate for up to 1 month.

PRO PREP TIP

If your mixture seems too dry, add a touch of extra-virgin olive oil to the mix in step 3 before spreading on the pan and baking.

Sweet-and-Salty Trail Mix

Yield: 4 portions

Prep Time: 15 minutes

Cook Time: 15 minutes

This snack is IRRESISTIBLE! You may want to divide this batch into even smaller portions to keep you from eating the entire thing in one day. Your house will smell amazing as the ingredients bake—bonus!

1 cup (110 g) roughly chopped raw pecans

1 cup (110 g) whole raw almonds

½ cup (55 g) whole raw cashews

½ cup (72 g) salted sunflower seeds

¾ cup (105 g) salted pumpkin seeds

½ cup (75 g) raisins

¼ teaspoon Himalayan pink salt

2 tablespoons (28 g) coconut oil

2 tablespoons (40 g) raw honey

1 teaspoon pure vanilla extract

1. Preheat the oven to 350°F (180°C). Line a large, rimmed baking sheet with parchment paper. Set aside.

2. In a large bowl, combine the pecans, almonds, cashews, sunflower and pumpkin seeds, raisins, and pink salt.

3. Place the coconut oil and honey in 2 separate small microwave-safe bowls and heat in the microwave for 20 seconds to melt.

4. Pour the melted coconut oil and honey, along with the vanilla, into the bowl with the nuts and seeds. Stir to combine until everything is coated. Spread the mixture onto the prepared baking sheet.

5. Bake for about 15 minutes, until the mix begins turning golden brown, stirring halfway through. Remove the baking sheet from the oven and allow the trail mix to cool in the pan for 5 to 10 minutes.

6. Equally divide the trail mix into 4 containers. Store in the refrigerator for up to 2 weeks.

Healthier Tuna Salad

Yield: 4 to 6 portions

Prep Time: 15 minutes

With a few swaps this tuna salad is the perfect food-prep snack or meal. Using avocado instead of mayonnaise boosts the nutrient value and makes it extra creamy. Enjoy this in whole grain pita bread or lettuce wraps or spreading on crackers or toast.

3 cans (5 ounces, or 142 g, each) tuna in water, drained

1 medium seedless cucumber, diced

2 large, ripe avocados, peeled, pitted, and sliced

1 small or medium red onion, diced

¼ cup (4 g) loosely packed chopped fresh cilantro (optional)

2 tablespoons (30 ml) fresh lime juice

Himalayan pink salt, to taste

Dash freshly ground black pepper

Extra-virgin olive oil, to taste

Whole wheat or super seed crackers, for serving (optional)

1. To a large bowl, add the tuna, cucumber, avocados, onion, cilantro, lime juice, pink salt, and black pepper. Mix together the ingredients while smashing the avocados to combine well.

2. Stir in a drizzle of olive oil a little bit at a time until the desired consistency is reached.

3. Equally divide the tuna salad into 4 to 6 containers. Store in the refrigerator for up to 2 days. When ready to enjoy, serve with the crackers (if using).

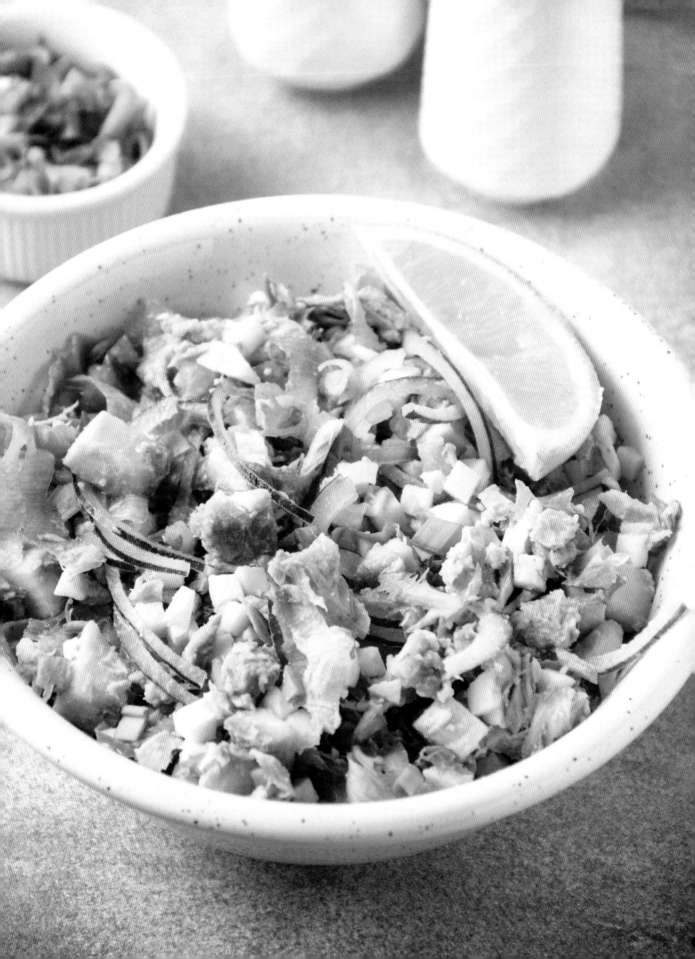

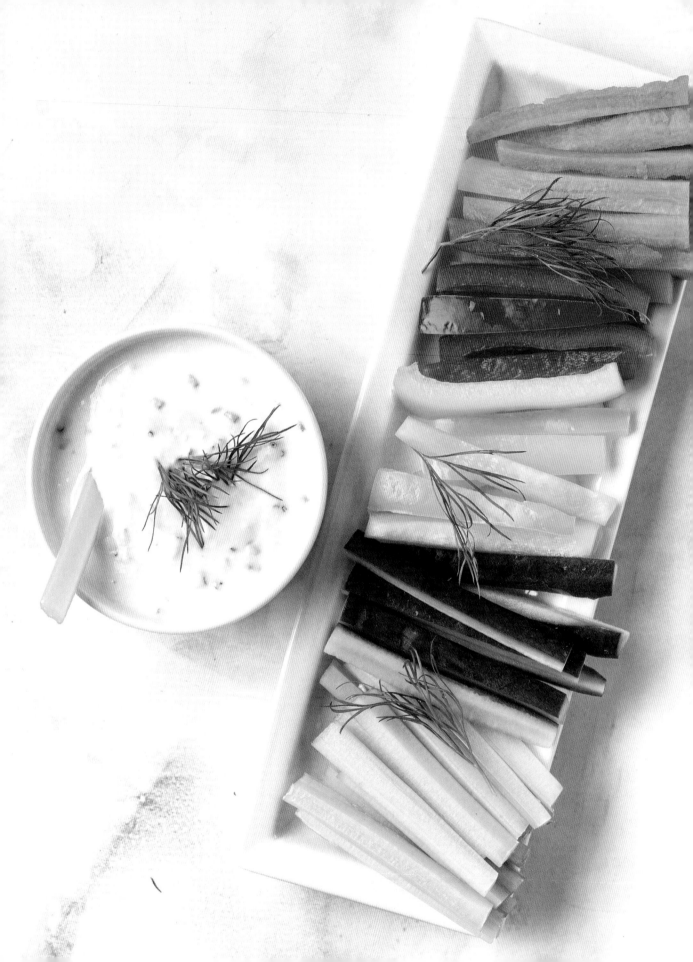

Vegetables with Greek Yogurt Dip

Yield: 4 portions

Prep Time: 15 minutes

You can find two other variations of this dip on page 138: Herb Greek Yogurt Dip and Spicy Greek Yogurt Dip.

VEGETABLES

3 large carrots, peeled and cut into sticks

2 large cucumbers, cut into sticks

2 cups (150 g) snap peas

1 pint (275 g) cherry tomatoes

1 large red bell pepper, cut into sticks

1 large yellow bell pepper, cut into sticks

YOGURT DIP

1 cup (240 g) plain Greek-style yogurt

1 seedless cucumber, grated

2 teaspoons fresh lemon juice

Dash sea salt

Few sprigs fresh dill, chopped

1. Equally divide the vegetables into 4 containers.

2. Mix together all the yogurt dip ingredients in a medium bowl and equally divide the dip into 4 small containers.

3. Store both the vegetables and yogurt dip in the refrigerator for up to 5 days.

Crispy Cubed Tofu

Whether you prefer Italian, Asian, or Mexican flavors, the great thing about cooking with tofu is its ability to take on the flavors of whatever you put with it. Tofu is best seasoned before (by marinating) or even during cooking. Once crispy, you can leave the tofu plain or season it with additional sauces, such as soy sauce or sesame oil.

Yield: 3 or 4 portions

Prep Time: 20 minutes

Cook Time: 5 minutes

1 package (14 to 16 ounces, or 392 to 454 g) extra-firm tofu

Himalayan pink salt, to taste

2 tablespoons (30 ml) extra-virgin olive oil

1. To remove the liquid from the block of tofu, you'll want to drain and press it. First, remove the tofu from its packaging and drain any liquid. Set the block of tofu onto a folded paper towel (you may want to put a plate underneath the paper towel to catch excess liquid). Set another folded paper towel on top of the block. Put a plate or small cutting board on top of the tofu and press down firmly to remove the liquid.

2. Remove the tofu from the paper towels and place on a cutting board. Cut the tofu into 1-inch (2.5 cm) cubes and pat dry with a paper towel if there is any remaining liquid. Season with the salt.

3. Heat the olive oil in a large skillet over medium-high heat. Once the oil begins to shimmer, add the tofu cubes without overcrowding the pan. When the undersides are golden brown, about 2 minutes, turn the cubes with silicone-handle tongs. Continue frying until all sides are browned and crispy, about 2 more minutes. Transfer to a cooling rack.

4. Equally divide the tofu cubes into 3 or 4 containers. Store in the refrigerator for up to 5 days. You can eat cold or warm; to reheat, warm in a skillet over medium heat for 2 to 3 minutes.

Superfood Popcorn

If you're anything like me, you love to snack! This superfood snack takes minutes to put together, and it's rich in protein, fiber, minerals, and vitamins.

Yield: 4 portions

Prep Time: 5 minutes

2 teaspoons spirulina powder

¼ cup (16 g) nutritional yeast

½ teaspoon garlic salt

4 cups (32 g) air-popped popcorn

Coconut oil spray

1. In a small bowl, mix together the spirulina powder, nutritional yeast, and garlic salt.

2. Spray the popcorn with the coconut oil spray. Pour the seasoning mix onto the popcorn and toss to coat.

3. Equally divide the popcorn into 4 containers. Store in a cool, dry place for up to 4 days.

Nut Butter Roll-Ups

This super-quick snack hardly takes any time to prep; however, if you want to take this with you and put it together at work, school, or on the road, check out step 3 below. This recipe uses bananas, but you can substitute apple slices or celery. Have fun trying different combinations!

Yield: 4 portions

Prep Time: 5 minutes

4 tablespoons (64 g) nut butter of choice

4 large (10 inches, or 25 cm, each) whole wheat tortillas

4 bananas

1. Spread 1 tablespoon (16 g) of nut butter onto each tortilla.

2. Place a banana on the outer edge of a tortilla and tightly roll it up. Slice the roll into 1-inch (2.5 cm) pieces.

3. If you are eating roll-ups the same day you make them, put the slices into containers. To have the ingredients ready a few days in advance, store the nut butter in small containers and the tortillas in resealable plastic bags. When ready to enjoy, assemble the roll-ups.

Roasted Vegetables

Roasting vegetables has become a regular part of my meal-prep routine. Because almost any vegetable can be roasted, feel free to experiment with your favorites. Use this recipe as a starting point and keep a couple things in mind: one, don't overcrowd the pan, and two, keep similar veggies together, such as root vegetables (potatoes, beets), cruciferous vegetables (cauliflower, brussels sprouts), and other vegetables (bell peppers, onion, tomatoes). Another great thing about roasting veggies is that the possibilities for repurposing them are endless. I like to use them in anything from pasta and omelets to wraps and rice. They are such a great way to include more vegetables in your diet!

Yield: 2 or 3 portions
Prep Time: 15 minutes
Cook Time: 1 hour

1 large sweet potato, unpeeled and cubed

1 cup (150 g) frozen cubed butternut squash

3 tablespoons (45 ml) extra-virgin olive oil

¼ cup (60 ml) balsamic vinegar

½ teaspoon dried thyme

½ teaspoon garlic salt

1 large yellow or white onion, sliced

1 large red bell pepper, cut into medium-size pieces

Coarse salt or Himalayan pink salt, to taste

Freshly ground black pepper, to taste

1. Preheat the oven to 375°F (190°C). Line 2 medium, rimmed baking sheets with parchment paper. Set aside.

2. In a large bowl, toss the sweet potato and squash with the olive oil, balsamic vinegar, thyme, and garlic salt. Evenly spread out the sweet potato and squash on one of the prepared baking sheets, reserving any extra marinade in the bowl. Cook for about 1 hour.

3. In the bowl with the reserved marinade, add the onion and bell pepper, and toss to coat. Evenly spread out the onion and bell pepper on the remaining prepared baking sheet. Cook for the last 30 minutes of the sweet potato–squash cooking time. Remove both pans from the oven, add the salt and pepper, and let the vegetables cool.

4. Equally divide the roasted vegetables into 2 or 3 containers. Store in the refrigerator for up to 5 days. To reheat, place the veggies on a baking sheet and warm in the oven at 350°F (180°C) for 4 to 5 minutes or warm them in a large skillet (without oil) over medium-high heat for 2 to 3 minutes, tossing frequently.

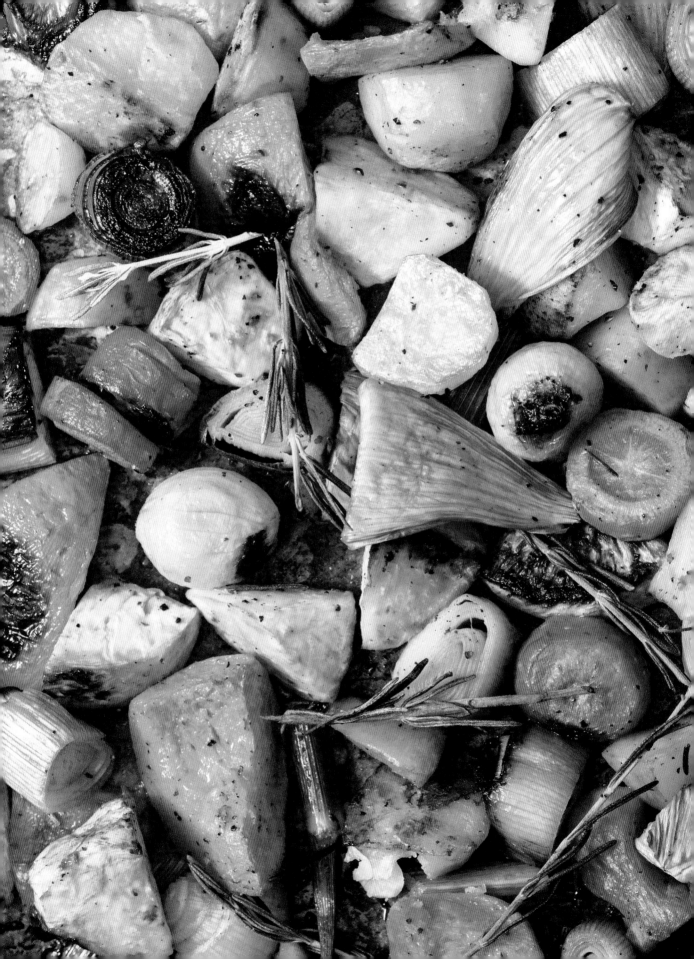

Cauliflower Rice

Feel free to add your favorite herbs, spices, or seasonings to make this recipe to your personal tastes.

Yield: 4 portions
Prep Time: 10 minutes
Cook Time: 5 minutes

1 head cauliflower, washed and roughly chopped

1 tablespoon (15 ml) olive oil

Himalayan pink salt, to taste

Freshly ground black pepper, to taste

1. Put the cauliflower in a food processor or blender, in 1-cup (70 g) batches, and pulse until rice-size pieces are reached.

2. Heat the olive oil in a large skillet over medium heat for 1 to 2 minutes. Add the riced cauliflower to the skillet and cook and stir for 4 to 5 minutes. Season with the pink salt and black pepper. Remove from the heat.

3. Equally divide the rice into 4 containers. Store in the refrigerator for up to 5 days.

Garlicky Green Beans

Ten minutes to deliciousness! Fresh green beans and garlic make this side dish unforgettable.

Yield: 3 or 4 portions
Prep Time: 10 minutes
Cook Time: 10 minutes

2 teaspoons extra-virgin olive oil, divided

1 pound (454 g) fresh green beans, ends trimmed

1 teaspoon Himalayan pink salt

1 teaspoon freshly ground black pepper

¼ cup (60 ml) water

3 garlic cloves, minced

1. Heat a large skillet with a lid over high heat. Add 1 teaspoon of the olive oil and the beans, salt, and pepper. Cook, turning the beans constantly, until they are bright green with some charred edges, 3 to 4 minutes.

2. Add the water, cover, and steam for 2 to 3 minutes. Remove the lid and stir the beans until the water has cooked off. Add the remaining 1 teaspoon oil and the garlic. Cook for 2 more minutes, stirring once or twice. Remove from the heat.

3. Equally divide into 3 or 4 containers. Store in the refrigerator for up to 5 days. To reheat, microwave for 1 to 2 minutes.

Crispy Sweet Potato Medallions

Yield: 4 to 6 portions

Prep Time: 15 minutes

Cook Time: 20 minutes

If you love sweet potato fries, then you will love this healthy homemade recipe. Lightly pan-frying the potatoes makes them crispier than cutting them into fries and baking them in the oven.

2 tablespoons (30 ml) extra-virgin olive oil, plus more if needed

4 medium sweet potatoes, peeled and sliced into ½-inch-thick (13 mm) rounds

1 teaspoon dried parsley

1 tablespoon (15 ml) Himalayan pink salt

1. Heat the olive oil in a large skillet over medium heat for 30 seconds. Add the potatoes to the skillet in one layer. Do not overcrowd the rounds. (Note: Depending on the size of your skillet, you may have to cook your potatoes in batches. Add a little more olive oil to the pan if necessary.) Stir to coat all the rounds with the oil. Add the parsley and salt, and mix well.

2. Cook the potatoes, stirring occasionally, for 15 to 20 minutes. Keep an eye on them so they don't burn, but make sure they get nice and crispy.

3. Remove the skillet from the heat when the potatoes are soft on the inside (you can easily pierce the medallions with a fork) but crispy on the outside. Place onto a plate lined with paper towels. Let the potatoes cool for 5 to 6 minutes.

4. Equally divide the medallions into 4 to 6 containers. Store in the refrigerator for up to 5 days. To reheat, warm in a skillet over medium-high heat for 3 minutes, turning once, or warm in the oven at 375°F (190°C) for 4 to 5 minutes.

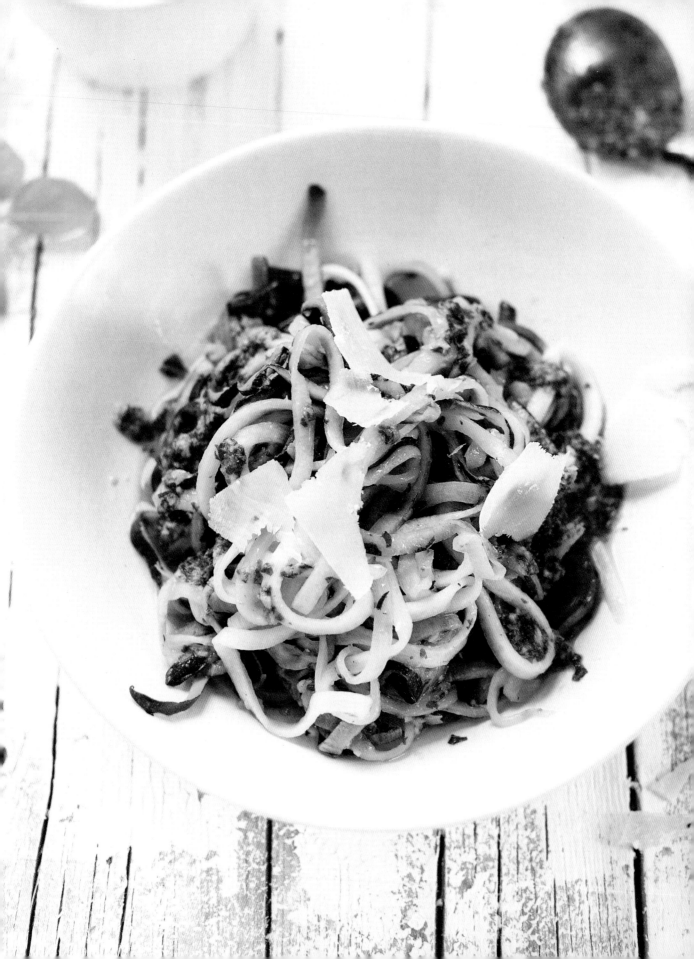

Pesto Zucchini Noodles

Yield: 4 portions

Prep Time: 15 minutes

Cook Time: 5 minutes

Zucchini noodles, zoodles, veggie spirals—they're great no matter what you call them. Zucchini noodles are fantastic cold and can be added to any salad. This recipe is meant to mimic spaghetti, and my homemade Pesto (page 137) is the perfect accompaniment.

3 medium zucchini, unpeeled

1 tablespoon (15 ml) extra-virgin olive oil

3 tablespoons (48 g) Pesto (page 137)

2 teaspoons Parmesan cheese, plus more for topping

1. Turn the zucchini into noodles. You can create zucchini noodles with a countertop spiralizer, a handheld spiralizer, or a Y vegetable peeler. If using a countertop spiralizer, cut off both ends of the zucchini, position it in the spiralizer, and turn the handle to make a beautiful pile of curly "noodles." With a handheld spiralizer, use it like a large pencil sharpener. Run a Y or julienne vegetable peeler down the entire length of the zucchini to create ribbon-like strands.

2. Heat the olive oil in a large skillet over medium heat for 30 seconds. Add the pesto to the pan and heat through. Add the zucchini noodles and cheese, using silicone-handle tongs to toss to coat the noodles in the pesto. Cook, turning the noodles frequently, for 3 to 4 minutes. Remove from the heat.

3. Equally divide the noodles into 4 containers and let cool before refrigerating. Store in the refrigerator for up to 3 days. To reheat, microwave for 30 to 45 seconds. Do not overheat.

Baked Tortilla Triangles

It is worth the extra couple minutes to prepare these "chips" on your own. Plus, you will save yourself more than half the calories and fat of store-bought chips.

Yield: 16 triangles

Prep Time: 5 minutes

Cook Time: 10 minutes

2 large (10 inches, or 25 cm, each) whole wheat tortillas

Nonstick cooking spray (olive, coconut, or avocado oil)

Chili powder, to taste

Garlic powder, to taste

Himalayan pink salt, to taste

1. Preheat the oven to 350°F (180°C).

2. On a cutting board, cut each tortilla in half and each half into 4 triangles.

3. Place the tortilla triangles on a large baking sheet. Do not overlap. Lightly spray both sides of the triangles with the cooking spray.

4. Sprinkle the triangles with the chili powder, garlic powder, and pink salt.

5. Bake until golden brown, 6 to 8 minutes. Watch the tortillas so they don't burn. Remove from the oven and let cool in the pan for 2 to 3 minutes; they will crisp up as they cool.

6. Equally divide the tortilla triangles into containers. Store in a cool, dry place for up to 3 days.

Roasted Chickpeas

Feel free to experiment with different spices here. Some of my savory favorites include cayenne pepper and grated Parmesan cheese; for a sweet bite, try a little ground cinnamon and stevia.

Yield: 2 or 3 portions
Prep Time: 10 minutes
Cook Time: 30 minutes

1 can (15 ounces, or 425 g) chickpeas

1 tablespoon (15 ml) extra-virgin olive oil

½ teaspoon garlic powder

¼ teaspoon sea salt

1. Preheat the oven to 400°F (200°C). Line a large, rimmed baking sheet with aluminum foil or parchment paper. Set aside.

2. Place the chickpeas in a colander and thoroughly rinse them with cold water. Use a clean dish cloth to pat the chickpeas dry.

3. Place the chickpeas, olive oil, garlic powder, and sea salt into a large resealable plastic bag, securely seal the bag, and shake to coat. Transfer the chickpeas to the prepared baking sheet, evenly spreading them out.

4. Roast for about 30 minutes, shaking the pan to move the chickpeas around 3 or 4 times. Remove the baking sheet from the oven and let the chickpeas cool in the pan.

5. Equally divide the roasted chickpeas into 2 or 3 containers. Store in the refrigerator for up to 5 days. They may start to get a little soft and less crispy after a few days.

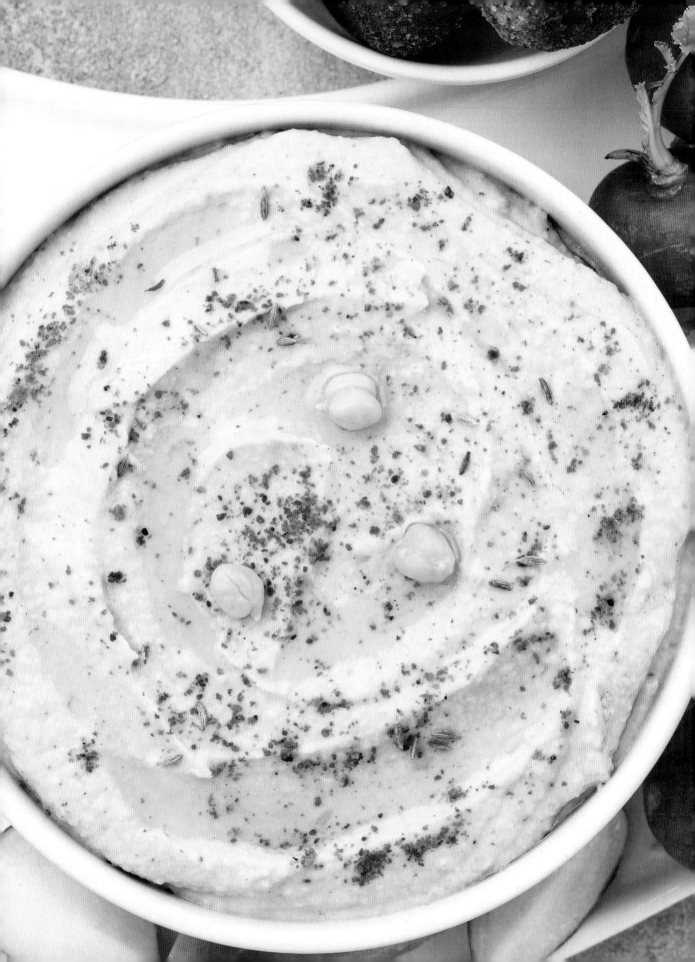

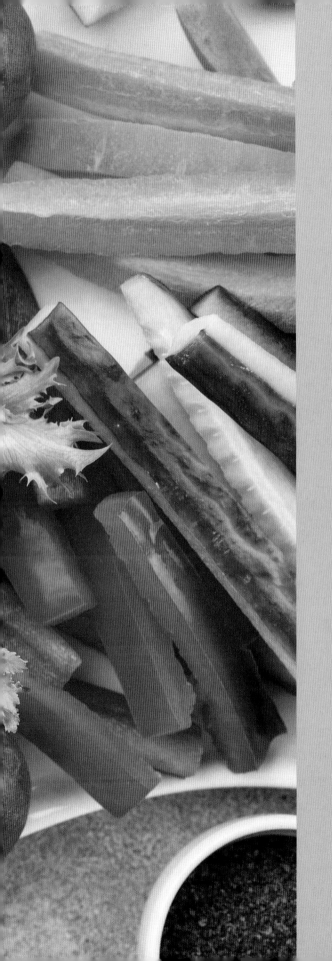
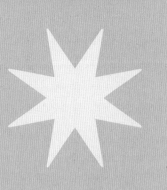
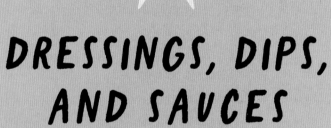

DRESSINGS, DIPS, AND SAUCES

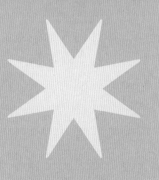
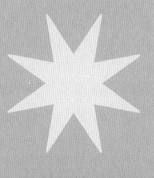

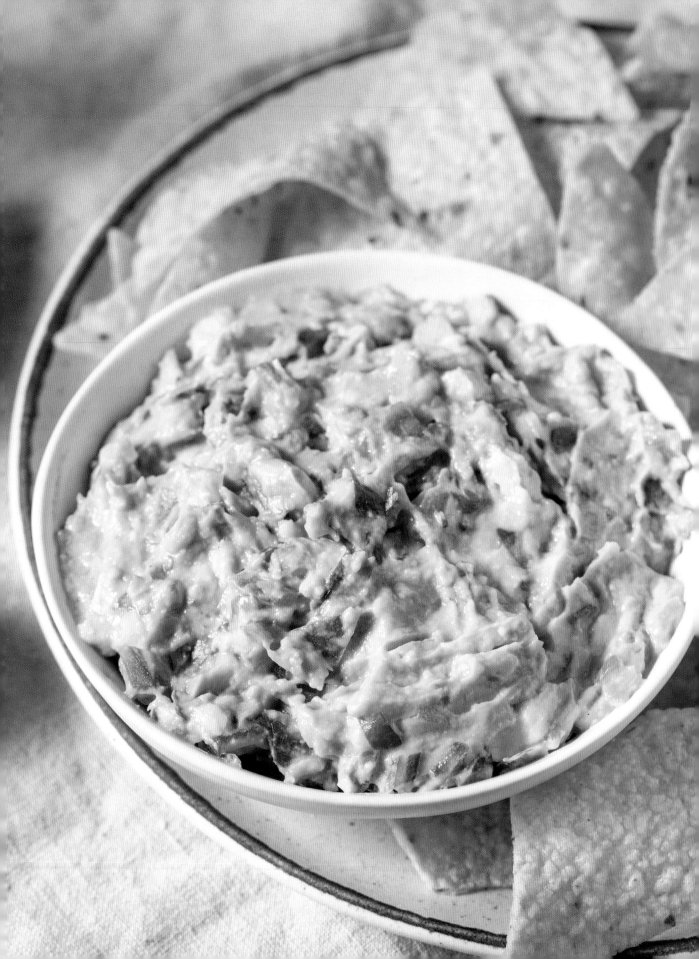

Guacamole

In 10 minutes, you can have fresh, healthy, and delicious guacamole that's better than any storebought version.

Yield: 4 or 5 portions

Prep Time: 10 minutes

4 large ripe avocados

1 cup (180 g) diced Roma tomatoes

½ teaspoon Himalayan pink salt

½ teaspoon cayenne pepper

½ teaspoon garlic powder

¼ cup (4 g) chopped fresh cilantro (optional)

½ cup (120 ml) fresh lime juice

1. Cut the avocados in half, carefully remove the pits, and use a spoon to scoop out the flesh. Place the flesh into a medium bowl. Mash the avocados with the back of a fork until the desired texture is achieved.

2. Add the tomatoes, pink salt, cayenne pepper, garlic powder, cilantro (if using), and lime juice. Stir to combine all the ingredients.

3. Equally divide the guacamole into 4 or 5 small containers. Before securing the lids, cover the guacamole with a small piece of plastic wrap. Gently press down so the wrap is touching the surface of the guacamole, then secure the lid. You may find a thin layer of discolored guacamole on top when reopening the container, but this layer should come off when you remove the plastic; if not, simply scrape it off with a knife before using. Store in the refrigerator for up to 4 days.

PRO PREP TIP

The riper the avocado, the easier it will be to turn it into guacamole. To select a ripe avocado, look for dark green skin, and then gently squeeze the avocado in the palm of your hand. If it's slightly soft (but not mushy), it's ripe enough to use right away.

Salsa

You can find this condiment on our table for breakfast, lunch, and dinner. Roma tomatoes are best for this recipe as they tend to be a "fleshier" and less watery tomato.

Yield: 4 or 5 portions

Prep Time: 15 minutes

4 Roma tomatoes, diced

½ small onion of choice, diced

2 garlic cloves, minced

1 to 2 tablespoons (1 to 2 g) chopped fresh cilantro

Himalayan pink salt, to taste

Freshly ground black pepper, to taste

Garlic powder, to taste

1. In a small bowl, add all the ingredients and combine. Stir with a spoon and mash a little—doing this will make the salsa juicy (as it sits, it will get even juicer).

2. Equally divide the salsa into 4 or 5 small containers. Store in the refrigerator for up to 5 days. (Note: If the salsa becomes watery after a few days, simply drain some of the liquid before eating.)

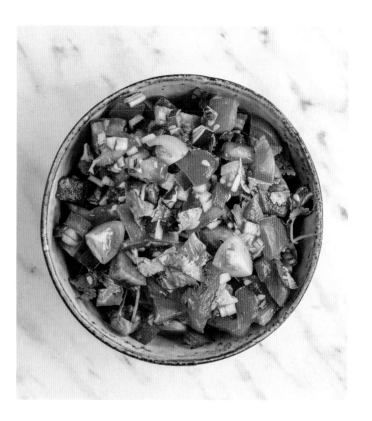

Avocado Aioli

Creamy, healthy, and beautiful . . . yes, please! Enjoy this deliciousness on sandwiches, wraps, potatoes, or anything barbecued.

Yield: 4 to 6 portions

Prep Time: 10 minutes

2 large ripe avocados

⅔ cup (160 g) low-fat plain Greek-style yogurt

½ teaspoon Himalayan pink salt

½ teaspoon garlic powder

½ teaspoon cayenne pepper

½ teaspoon crushed red pepper flakes

¼ cup (60 ml) fresh lime juice

1. Cut the avocados in half, carefully remove the pits, and use a spoon to scoop out the flesh. Place the flesh into a food processor or blender. Add all the remaining ingredients to the food processor or blender and blend until just smooth.

2. Equally divide the aioli into 4 to 6 small containers. Store in the refrigerator for up to 3 days.

3-Step Tomato Sauce

All you need is a few ingredients, a blender, a large pot, and 40 minutes to create a delicious meal. This fresh sauce is perfect for your favorite whole-grain pasta.

Yield: 5½ cups (48 ounces, or 1.4 kg)

Prep Time: 15 minutes

Cook Time: 25 minutes

6 cups (1.1 kg) roughly chopped fresh Roma tomatoes (about 17 tomatoes)

1 medium yellow onion, quartered

6 garlic cloves, peeled

½ cup (120 ml) extra-virgin olive oil

2 teaspoons sea salt

2 teaspoons dried oregano

1. Place all the ingredients into a high-speed blender and blend until smooth. The mixture will look a little pink at this point.

2. Pour the mixture into a large heavy-bottomed pot with a lid. Bring it to a simmer over medium heat, then reduce the heat to low to maintain a slow simmer for 15 to 20 minutes. Remove from the heat and let cool.

3. Store in an airtight container in the refrigerator for up to 4 or 5 days or freeze for up to 3 months.

Hummus

You'll never regret making your own hummus—it is so much tastier than store-bought varieties. Once you have this simple recipe down, experiment with ingredients like roasted red peppers, sun-dried tomatoes, curry, or cumin. If you don't have tahini, try substituting natural almond butter.

Yield: 6 portions

Prep Time: 10 minutes

1 can (15 ounces, or 425 g) chickpeas, drained and rinsed

3 to 5 tablespoons (45 to 75 ml) fresh lemon juice

1½ tablespoons (25 g) tahini

2 garlic cloves, minced

½ teaspoon salt of choice

2 tablespoons (30 ml) extra-virgin olive oil

1. Place all the ingredients in a blender (in the order they are listed) and blend until smooth.

2. Equally divide the hummus into 6 small containers. Store in the refrigerator for up to 5 days.

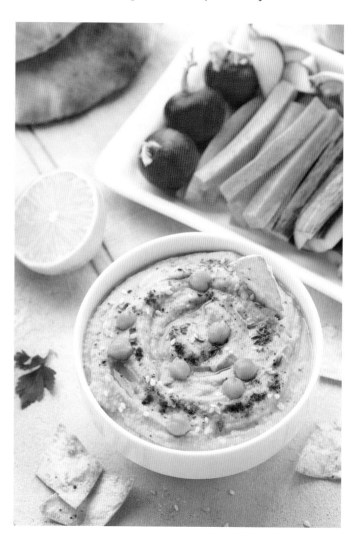

Pesto

Pesto is one of my favorite flavors. I love it on pasta, pizza, and in dips. It's not always easy to find store-bought pesto with clean ingredients, and it can be expensive. This simple recipe is a must-try!

Yield: About 1 cup (260 g)

Prep Time: 10 minutes

2 cups (80 g) loosely packed fresh basil leaves

3 garlic cloves

½ cup (50 g) freshly grated Parmesan cheese

⅓ cup (80 ml) extra-virgin olive oil

¼ cup (34 g) pine nuts (you can substitute walnuts if pine nuts are hard to find)

1. Add all the ingredients to a food processor or blender and process until almost smooth.

2. Store in an airtight container in the refrigerator for up to 7 days or in the freezer for up to 6 months.

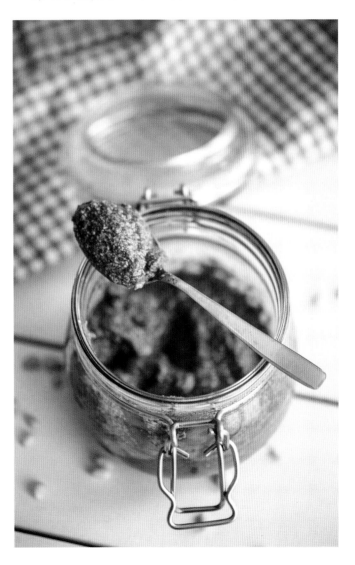

Greek Yogurt Dips

Healthy store-bought dips are a rare find; instead, whip together a few clean ingredients to create delicious and inexpensive multipurpose dips. No one will be the wiser.

Yield: 2 to 4 portions

Prep Time: 10 minutes

SPICY GREEK YOGURT DIP

2 cups (480 g) low-fat plain Greek-style yogurt

1 garlic clove, minced

½ cup (120 g) Salsa (page 134)

2 tablespoons (30 ml) fresh lime juice

2 teaspoons (4 g) chili powder

½ teaspoon cayenne pepper

2 teaspoons (4 g) cumin

½ teaspoon paprika

Salt of choice, to taste

HERB GREEK YOGURT DIP

¾ cup (180 g) low-fat plain Greek-style yogurt

1 garlic clove, minced

2 tablespoons (2 g) chopped chives

¼ teaspoon salt of choice

¼ teaspoon freshly ground black pepper

¼ teaspoon dried dill

1 tablespoon (15 ml) fresh lemon juice

FRUIT DIP DELIGHT

3 cups (720 g) low-fat plain Greek-style yogurt

1 scoop vanilla whey protein powder

½ cup (120 g) natural creamy almond or peanut butter

3 tablespoons pure maple syrup

1 teaspoon pure vanilla extract

Dash ground cinnamon

TO MAKE SPICY GREEK YOGURT DIP

1. Place all the ingredients into a medium bowl and stir until well combined.

2. Equally divide into 4 small containers. Store in the refrigerator for up to 3 days.

TO MAKE HERB GREEK YOGURT DIP

1. Place all the ingredients into a small bowl and stir until well combined.

2. Equally divide into 2 small containers. Store in the refrigerator for up to 3 days.

TO MAKE FRUIT DIP DELIGHT

1. Add all the ingredients to a medium bowl and whisk together until well combined. The dip should be smooth and creamy.

2. Equally divide into 2 small containers and top each one with a sprinkle of cinnamon. Store in the refrigerator for up to 3 days.

Salad Dressings

I often get asked about healthy dressings for salads. I just have one rule: make your own. Doing this is easy and inexpensive, and you have control over the ingredients you're putting in your food, since store-bought dressings can be laden with additives, sugar, and unhealthy fats. Here are three of my favorite recipes so you can start making your own. It's fun to experiment with additional ingredients to suit your taste preferences and "dress up" any salad.

Yield: 4 portions

Prep Time: 5 minutes

BASIC SALAD DRESSING

⅓ cup (80 ml) extra-virgin olive oil

⅓ cup (80 ml) balsamic vinegar

1 scant teaspoon roasted garlic and bell pepper seasoning

CITRUS SALAD DRESSING

¼ cup (60 ml) extra-virgin olive oil

2 tablespoons (30 ml) raw apple cider vinegar

3 tablespoons (12 g) nutritional yeast

Juice of 1 lemon

¼ teaspoon Himalayan pink salt

TANGY SALAD DRESSING

2 tablespoons (30 ml) red wine vinegar

2 teaspoons Dijon mustard

½ teaspoon sea salt

Freshly ground black pepper, to taste

½ cup (120 ml) extra-virgin olive oil

TO MAKE BASIC SALAD DRESSING

1. Add all the ingredients to a Mason jar or sealable container, secure the lid, and shake until well combined.

2. Equally divide the dressing into 4 containers. Store in the refrigerator for up to 5 days.

TO MAKE CITRUS SALAD DRESSING

1. Add all the ingredients to a Mason jar or sealable container, secure the lid, and shake until well combined.

2. Equally divide the dressing into 4 containers. Store in the refrigerator for up to 5 days.

TO MAKE TANGY SALAD DRESSING

1. Whisk together the vinegar, Dijon mustard, sea salt, and black pepper in a small bowl. Gradually whisk in the olive oil until well combined.

2. Equally divide the dressing into 4 containers. Store in the refrigerator for up to 1 week.

index

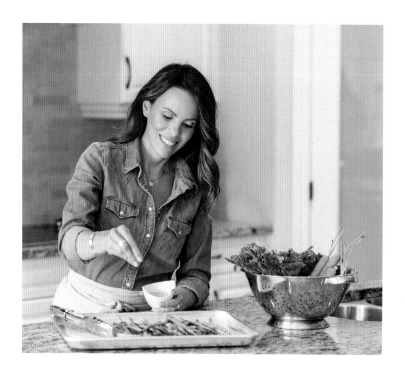

about the author

ERIN ROMEO is a nutrition coach, expert meal planner, and food-prep specialist. She's an advocate for good nutrition and regularly shares her tips and tricks for healthy eating on Instagram, where she's better known as the "foodprepprincess."

Erin connects with people around the globe from her home in Ontario, Canada, where she lives with her husband and young daughter. She's still as passionate about helping others get healthy, get organized, and get the results they want as she was with her first client ten years ago.

Erin and her meal preps have been featured online, including on Shape, The Kitchn, Daily Burn, BuzzFeed, and Brit+Co, and in *Oxygen* magazine. Her Instagram was voted one of the Best Meal Prep Accounts on Instagram by PopSugar.

Find out more at foodprepprincess.com and on Instagram @foodprepprincess.